THE TOKYO DIET

THE TOKYO DIET

by Dr. Yoko I. Takahashi
with
Bruce Cassiday

CREATED BY BILL ADLER

William Morrow and Company, Inc.

New York

Library of Congress Cataloging in Publication Data

Takahashi, Yoko I.
  The Tokyo diet.

  Includes index.
  1. Reducing diets—Recipes. 2. Cookery, Japanese.
I. Cassiday, Bruce. II. Title.
RM222.2.T27 1985   641.5'635   84-22752
ISBN 0-688-02865-9

Printed in the United States of America

  2 3 4 5 6 7 8 9 10

BOOK DESIGN BY JAMES UDELL

CONTENTS

PART ONE:
The Tokyo Diet

Chapter 1

THE FIVE FUNDAMENTALS

By following their own philosophy of life—to live in harmony with nature—the Japanese people have devised a built-in method of maintaining weight control through diet. The basic elements in this ingenious food regimen have been extracted to serve as a keystone for "The Tokyo Diet," with particular emphasis on five principles:

- What to eat
- How to prepare it
- How to serve it
- How to eat it
- What *not* to eat

WHAT TO EAT—JAPANESE-STYLE

Living in the limited totality of an island environment, the Japanese were obliged to improvise a method of survival by growing vital foodstuffs on tiny plots of earth or by capturing food live from the seas around them. Thus the primary sources of food in Japan come from what nature can provide:

- fish
- shellfish
- seaweed
- poultry
- vegetables
- beans
- fruit
- rice

Including tea, the national beverage, practically all the food eaten in Japan is produced locally, at least until recently. Today the Japanese eat a great deal of beef, but the traditional Japanese diet had little beef and little poultry.

It should be obvious to any dieter that to eat only fish, shellfish, seaweed, poultry, vegetables, beans, fruit, and rice is going to discourage excess weight gain—and in fact it *does* do so.

The key factor in the traditional Japanese diet is the restriction—by the environment and the availability of foodstuffs—to weight-control items. Note that there are several staples familiar to a Westerner missing from the diet mentioned above:

- bread
- dairy products, including cheese
- baked goods

HOW TO PREPARE IT—JAPANESE-STYLE

Equal in importance to the natural restriction to weight-control items is the Japanese method of food preparation.

THE TOKYO DIET

Living in harmony with nature, the Japanese cook tries to select only those foodstuffs that are in season, and to prepare them for consumption with as little alteration as possible.

The Japanese way is not to overcook. If anything, it is to serve food *al dente*—crunchy, tasty, and almost raw. The theory is that too much cooking destroys not only the structure of the natural product, but boils away the juices and nutrients that are essential to its taste and health benefits.

From a standpoint of weight control, there is another factor that is quite important. The Japanese chef does not like to cook meats that are heavy in fat. Every attempt is made to trim off all fat before any item is cooked.

A third point cannot be overstressed: The average serving of a course in a Japanese meal is only about one half of a Western portion. Again, this habit of skimping is the Japanese prerogative of preserving harmony between environment and population. If the environment is exploited by overplanting, overhunting, overfishing, there will be no food left. Serving small portions makes a little food go a long way, to preserve not only the land and the population, but the peace and harmony between each.

This is a very modern concept to civilized people in other lands but for centuries it was part of the Japanese philosophy of life.

As for *ways* of cooking food, the traditional Japanese methods favor preservation of taste and prevention of loss of nutrients. The Japanese prefer to:

- Steam their vegetables
- Stir-fry food in a saucepan
- Broil food spitted on a skewer or on a grill
- Boil vegetables and meats in such a way that the natural juices are preserved
- Fry food lightly, using unsaturated fats or oils

All these light cooking methods favor weight control because they are methods that never depend on gravies.

HOW TO SERVE IT—JAPANESE-STYLE

As the food is prepared, so is it served—as close to its natural state as possible. In other words, string beans are served fresh and green, appealing both to the palate and to the eye. Saltwater fish can be served uncooked in certain dishes. Vegetables can be served raw in salads or cooked lightly in vegetable dishes.

Color has a great deal to do with the way in which dishes are arranged when presented. Geometric patterns, designs, and art forms are as important as color—anything to make the appearance of the food on the dish a thing of beauty and harmony.

It is obvious that an artistic representation of a red circle of tomato, a pink placement of shrimp, a green piece of lettuce, and a purple portion of seaweed will be ruined by applying a heavy amount of French dressing indiscriminately all over the top. To keep foodstuffs at or near their natural state, the Japanese cook does not inundate salads with dressing, or meats and vegetables with heavy gravies.

When a condiment or sauce is used, it is often served on the side in a separate dish, so that the diner can dip a portion of food into the sauce.

Note what is being observed here. Gravies, dressings, and rich sauces in Western diets put on weight. Without any need to disguise the taste, or lack of it, in the basic ingredient being served, the Japanese cook can forgo the use of heavily seasoned and spiced condiments. If such delicacies are served on the side, they tend to be used more discriminatingly than when they are poured on top of the food.

HOW TO EAT IT—JAPANESE-STYLE

The pace of a Japanese meal is quite different from the pace of a Western meal. The typical American rushes pell-mell into a fast-food shop, orders a hamburger and fries, gobbles them up when they come, slaps down his money, and leaves in a rush. Even patrons in a high-priced restaurant are usually in a hurry, frantically signaling for the waiter to bring the next course or the bill. Eating United States-style is an exercise in desperation.

Exactly the opposite is true of the Japanese meal. Again, it is the harmony of nature that is important to the diner. In turn, etiquette developed over centuries of eating dictates that a meal should be eaten as slowly and carefully as it was prepared. Because the portions are small, each is eaten more slowly than a large piece would be. Because the food has been prepared in as natural a state as possible, it should be savored thoroughly. Because the course has been put together with an eye to aesthetics, the beauty of the placement should be enjoyed as the food is slowly eaten.

In fact, the longer a diner takes to eat a meal, the more satisfied the body is. Food bolted down is hardly noticed as it disappears from the plate. Food savored as it is eaten and enjoyed over quiet conversation and peaceful contemplation is much more thoroughly appreciated. When the body is in a state of repose and tranquillity, it can absorb food and extract its energy much easier than food that is taken in under stress.

Note that the way the Japanese people eat a meal tends to control weight. There is no gobbling and little chance of eating past satiation. One tends to eat only as much as one needs in slower-motion dining.

WHAT *NOT* TO EAT—JAPANESE-STYLE

The traditional Japanese diet, developed over centuries of self-discipline and harmony with nature, is remarkable not especially for what it features but for what it *lacks*. By and large, the items it lacks are those that provide the highest caloric intake for Americans.

For example, the traditional Japanese diet did not contain any bread or baked goods made from grains. Small cakes and sweets were prepared for eating—but none was actually made as important a part of the meal as bread was for peoples in the rest of the world.

Dairy products also were missing traditionally from the Japanese diet. Not only did the Japanese never drink cow's milk, but they never used butter on bread—having neither—nor did they ever use much cheese or cheese products in their diet.

Baked goods—aside from bread—were never featured as they were (and are) in Western diets. Cakes, pies, pastries, puddings, cookies, and so on, were simply not used for desserts or snacks.

As has been noted, there were also few gravies. Nor were dressings and sauces made to be poured over the top of vegetables or meats.

Obviously, the list of food items lacking from the traditional Japanese diets points up one fact: What the Japanese did not eat were those foods that cause the most trouble to non-Japanese people suffering from overweight or from the effects of self-indulgence.

THE TOKYO DIET IN TRANSITION

Although today there may be little time for aesthetics in eating—at least you would think so, the way people rush into and out of fast-food shops everywhere—the basics of a traditional weight-control diet from the past remain in the Japanese way of eating and provide a time-tested method to fight overweight and trim the body.

In Japan the tea ceremony survives with its simulation of a rippling stream in the bubbling sound of the teapot. This custom was developed centuries ago to provide a subtle experience uniting humankind and nature through serenity, beauty, and inner contemplation as the tea was drunk and the food accompanying it was eaten.

Even the memory of the samurai survives, his dedication to the martial arts, to preserving peace, not creating strife, living so as to permit the rest of his kinfolk to exist in harmony with nature.

But these are only pale memories of a more vigorous past.

Tokyo today is Westernized, with fast-food shops, pizza parlors, and junk food on sale everywhere. More and more the urban Japanese prefer dry cereal or toast and eggs for breakfast rather than the traditional rice and soup. Bread with butter or margarine is steadily increasing in popularity. Western dairy products are slowly supplementing the basic staples—rice, vegetables, and fish. Poultry sales have shot up 1,000 percent in the past twenty years. Hamburgers are now the favorite food of the young!

The protein intake of the average Japanese is equivalent to that of the average American. The Japanese ingest a smaller percentage of Calories from fats than Americans do, with a diet that is nutritionally better balanced. However, there are now some Japanese children who are seriously overweight—a problem that did not even exist in Japan fifty years ago.

Yet the basics of good eating are present in the traditional Japanese diet. They have been extracted and presented here in The Tokyo Diet, and they can easily be followed by anyone who wants to practice intelligent weight control.

Why not you?

Chapter 2

THE U.S. DIETARY GUIDELINES

During the years after World War II, government nutritionists in America became more and more concerned over the growing number of heart attacks, the increase in heart disease, and the general flabbiness of the American people. In February 1980 a 20-page publication titled *Nutrition and Your Health—Dietary Guidelines for Americans* was issued by the U.S. Departments of Agriculture and Health, Education and Welfare.

The study confirmed what many nutritionists already knew: that there *was* a correlation between overweight and the consumption of more Calories than a person needed; and that there was a relationship between heart attacks and eating too many foods high in saturated fat, which caused buildups of cholesterol in the blood vessels.

The publication suggested that diet had a great deal to do with health and that certain changes should be made in the typical diet to make Americans healthier. One of the key points made in the study was a reiteration of an ancient axiom known even to the Greeks:

Moderation in eating is the best guide to maintain health.

But there were at least five more points in the study that were important, at least to anyone who might be familiar with what went into a typical Japanese diet:

- Maintain an ideal weight at all times.
- Eat a variety of foods.
- Eat foods with adequate starch and fiber.
- Avoid too much fat, saturated fat, and cholesterol.
- Avoid too much sugar.

Let's take up those points one by one:

MAINTAINING AN IDEAL WEIGHT

The government scientists came up with several important points to keep weight under control, that is, at a healthful minimum. The pointers were somewhat obvious, but in need of reiteration:

- Cut back on serving sizes.
- Cut down on fats, sugars, and alcohol.
- Exercise more.

The most arresting pointer was the first: "Cut back on serving sizes."

As noted in Chapter 1, as a general rule the quantity of each portion in a Japanese meal is about half the amount one would serve in a Western meal. Japan is small, and arable land is limited. By consuming too much, many people would starve. By consuming less, they can all live healthy lives.

In America the opposite is true. It is a land of great plenty, of bountiful resources, of huge supplies of food. The more you have, the more you eat.

The second pointer in the U.S. guidelines for maintaining an ideal weight is to cut down on fats and sugars. That too might come right out of a traditional Japanese diet. Meat is prepared and eaten lean, that is, all the fat is cut off at the start.

Nor is animal fat used to cook in the Japanese manner. The oil used is vegetable oil. This type of oil makes food cooked in it much lighter, and it does not solidify even when the food cools. Besides, it is healthier than animal fat. In any case, cooking oil is used only slightly, and most food is not fried for long.

As for sugar, it does not appear in rich pastries or in pies or cakes as it does in the average American dessert. Dessert in Japan is more apt to be simply a fresh or preserved piece of fruit or melon.

EATING A VARIETY OF FOODS FOR GOOD HEALTH

The government nutritionists also recommended a large variety of foodstuffs—fruits of all kinds; vegetables, breads, and cereals; dairy products; and meat, fish, and poultry products—to make the American diet more wide-ranging. The idea was to include all the vitamins and minerals needed for good health in such a way that these essential ingredients did not all come from the same food day after day.

Selection of different foods from within each group of foodstuffs—fruits, vegetables, cereals, and meats—would increase the range of nutrients and make the diner healthier.

There were four main rules to follow:

- Eat more fruits.
- Eat more vegetables.

- Eat not only dark green vegetables but starchy vegetables and dried bean dishes.
- Use more grain products, especially whole grains.

These four rules are, of course, right out of Japanese tradition too. The melons and fruits, the green vegetables, the starchy vegetables, and the many different kinds of dishes derived from the soybean: Not only is there variety in their tastes, but in their shapes and sizes and colors as well.

And rice—that's special all by itself. Rice is served at every Japanese meal. Actually, the government nutritionists seemed to be telling the American people to eat in a more Japanese way!

EATING FOODS WITH STARCH AND FIBER

The government nutritionists were also trying to persuade the American people to use more starch and fiber in their diets. The theory was that the typical American diet contained too many fats and sweets and not enough good solid hard foods.

Those used to eating fat-filled foods and easy-to-chew sweets were losing their taste for the more natural fruits, vegetables, and whole-grain foods. People addicted to processed foods and too many meat dishes were being babied; they were getting their Calories in concentrated form but were missing out on an ingredient essential to their health—namely, fiber.

Several main points were made:

- Eat fruits and vegetables rather than fats and sweets.
- Eat potatoes, sweet potatoes, yams, peas, and dried beans more often.

19

- Emphasize whole-grain cereal products—brown rice, oatmeal, and whole-wheat cereals and breads.

There are several reasons high-fiber foods help you fight excess weight:

- The simple fact is that the more fiber you eat, the fewer Calories you consume. Fibrous foods, particularly fruits and vegetables, usually provide few Calories.
- Fiber absorbs water as it travels through the digestive tract. In filling up, it bulks out and fills the stomach, making you less hungry.
- It takes longer to chew foods with fiber in them. Chewing slows down the process of eating, making it more leisurely and calming.
- Chewing longer on the food you eat makes you feel as if you are eating a great deal rather than a small amount, and it satisfies your hunger.

For all the good it does, Calorie-counting sometimes forms the wrong habits for diet-conscious people. By counting the high caloric content of starchy foods like potatoes, breads, and grains, dieters tend to avoid these foods as "fattening." But starch is no more fattening than any other food element. And it has been learned that starch and fiber are both necessary ingredients in a wholesome diet.

The Japanese provide more fruits and vegetables in their diet than Americans do. The Japanese diet includes vegetables like yams, potatoes, and peas, plus dried beans. In Japan they don't use maize (what Americans call "corn"). But the Japanese often eat buckwheat in noodle form; and they eat rice, a grain food, at every meal, as stated before.

Here is a diet that has plenty of starch and fiber already in it!

AVOIDING TOO MUCH FAT, SATURATED FAT, AND CHOLESTEROL

The government's nutritional study found that the immoderate consumption of fats, saturated fat and cholesterol, and excess sodium were beginning to be named as the main reasons for the high incidence of heart disease in the American people.

The insidious damage to the blood vessels caused by the intake of saturated fat and cholesterol was a fairly recent discovery; not only did it contribute to overweight, but it helped produce heart disease. High levels of blood cholesterol—obtained through certain foodstuffs—was found to lead to atherosclerosis, or hardening of the arteries. This was the underlying problem that caused most heart and blood vessel diseases.

It was also discovered that most of the fat, saturated fat, and cholesterol come from animal fats and oils, meat, poultry, egg yolks, and dairy products.

Of course, one of the most obvious differences between Japanese and American cookery is the lack of dairy products like butter, cheese, and milk. Nine important pointers were given by the government report in its discussion on saturated fat and cholesterol:

- Select lean hamburger and lean roasts, chops, and steaks, trimmed of fat.
- Drain all meat drippings.
- Limit the amount of margarine or other fats used on bread and vegetables.

- Emphasize low-fat and skimmed milk instead of whole milk.
- Cut down on the amount of fat used in recipes, added to foods in cooking, and at the table.
- Limit the number of fried foods, especially breaded or batter-fried.
- Moderate the amounts of organ meats and egg yolks in the diet.
- Use fewer creamed foods and rich desserts in the menu.
- Watch the amount of salad dressing used.

These random points might almost come out of the traditional Japanese menu. One especially interesting cooking technique is the Japanese cook's habit of often cutting off poultry skin and the fat underneath it before cooking; this is an obvious way to cut down on fat content and to give the diner a proper bite-size portion to grip with chopsticks.

AVOIDING TOO MUCH SUGAR

The government nutritionists found that one of the most obvious villains in any weight-watching program was sugar. Although carbohydrates were a vigorous source of immediate energy in the form of Calories, sugar gave the eater little more than a quick lift. It did not have any nutritional pluses—no vitamins, no potassium, no calcium, no protein, no iron, and so on.

Sugar also tended to add weight when sufficient Calories were not used up by the body. Such caloric intake was stored in the body as fat rather than as muscle. For that reason, the intake of sugar, next to the intake of fat, was considered a major source of overweight. To be prudent, a person concerned about weight should avoid sugar whenever and wherever possible.

Carbohydrates existed in foodstuffs other than sugar—fruits and vegetables that provided many other important nutritional elements as well as carbohydrates. By depriving oneself of sugar, one did not cut out a primary source of quick energy.

Nutritionists said there were four good ways to decrease the amount of sugar consumed:

- Avoid sugar entirely and cut down on all artificially sweetened foods.
- Limit the amounts of sugar, jams, jellies, and syrups used in your diet.
- Reduce the amount of sugar in recipes for baked goods and desserts.
- Use fresh fruit or canned fruits packed in juice or light syrup rather than in heavy sugar syrup.

The Japanese use sugar when they can but in moderation—a teaspoonful here, a teaspoonful there. They do not put sugar in tea at all. They do not have jams, jellies, or preserves—because there is nothing to spread them on. The Japanese do not use baked goods the way the rest of the world does. Most of the sugar in their diet is natural—from fresh or canned fruits—exactly as recommended by the U.S. nutritional study.

HOW TO USE THE DIETARY GUIDELINES

We have discussed the dietary guidelines in some detail because of their striking similarity to the guidelines used by the traditional Japanese cook in preparing menus and in creating recipes for dishes. Somehow, it seemed to us that the Japanese got there first and organized much of their cuisine around the more salient points indicated in the United States dietary guidelines.

This may be an exaggeration, but if it is, the exaggeration is based on several important facts:

- The Japanese eat about one half the amount of food that we eat at one sitting.
- The Japanese prepare food for eating in as close to the natural state as possible.
- The Japanese diet includes a number of low-Calorie foods: vegetables, fruits, fish, and rice.
- The Japanese diet excludes a number of high-Calorie foods: butter, pastries, cheeses, gravies, sauces, and cooked desserts.

Are we saying you should immediately throw out all your recipe books featuring continental cuisine and American dishes and start eating strictly Japanese?

Not at all.

We are suggesting you experiment a little. Experimentation comes in several distinct steps, outlined below. The rest of the book will take you through these steps as you prepare to lose weight using what we call The Tokyo Diet, which is essentially the Japanese way of eating.

(1) Begin to *think* of food as the Japanese do.

- Think of it as something to be savored and enjoyed.
- Consider it something to be eaten with care and with contentment.
- Enjoy its flavor and its variety, not just its overall content.

(2) Try a Japanese dish now and then.

- It's probably best not to eat Japanese from morning to night at first.
- Try a well-known Japanese dish like *sukiyaki* or *tempura* at first.
- Practice eating rice and *sukiyaki* with chopsticks. It's an experience.

(3) Prepare your own traditional dishes in the Japanese way.

- Cook them in their most natural state.
- Do not add thick sauces, dressings, or relishes unless they are low in fat, salt, and sugar.

(4) Serve your own traditional dishes in the Japanese manner.

- Serve all food as attractively as possible in artistic and imaginative patterns.
- Use lots of natural garnishes for contrasting colors and shapes.
- Do not serve too much food; it is a temptation to overeat. If the food isn't there, you won't be able to finish it off.

Obviously, you aren't going to be able to make a total change in diet overnight—it's too great a culture shock. The best thing to do is to start small, by making one change in your diet, possibly substituting one Japanese-type dish you enjoy already for a rich casserole or meat dish. When you've adjusted to that change, move on to another one.

Don't push yourself too hard. The problem with most

diets is that they insist on strict adherence in order to guarantee results. Because of the tight strictures of such a diet, you begin to resist, and once you've lost the weight, you go right back to your old way of eating.

On the contrary, the important thing is to make small changes, but keep them consistent. Don't be satisfied by making one minor change in your diet—say, eating fewer rich salad dressings. Go a step further, and restructure the salads themselves. Then go on to vegetable dishes using the same foodstuffs in a new way.

We are not going to advise you to change your whole diet style and eat only vegetables, rice, and fish. Far from it. But you should begin to *think* about cooking from the Japanese point of view—a minimum of cooking, care in preparation of food, extra care in its serving.

Take the good dietary elements of the Japanese way and blend them with the best dietary elements of the American way. Then you'll have the perfect diet!

The Tokyo Diet.

Chapter 3

THE ART OF EATING LESS

The Japanese eat quite a bit less food than Americans do, yet each meal has a great many more courses and dishes than an American meal. The seeming contradiction lies in the fact that the Japanese diner eats extremely small portions of each food served.

This is a habit that helps keep food intake down and weight off.

RICE AND SOUP FOR BREAKFAST?

For example, here is a typical Japanese breakfast—which seems to be huge but really isn't when you break it down item by item.

Traditionally, it starts out with a bowl of rice (equivalent to a Westerner's morning buttered toast, dry cereal, or pancakes and never missing from any Japanese meal), and a bowl of soup. Although rice is always a separate item in a meal, it is often served with *nori* (dried laver, a type of seaweed). The *nori* comes in dried sheets. To eat *nori* and rice, the diner picks up a sheet with a pair of chopsticks and skillfully wraps a bite-size portion of rice in it.

For breakfast the soup is always *miso* soup. *Miso* soup is a type of thick, heavy potage called *misoshiru*. *Miso* is fermented soybean paste; it gives the soup its flavor.

The soup is composed of *dashi*, Japanese soup stock, plus a tablespoonful of *miso*. To this may be added a cube or so of *tofu*, soybean curd. In addition, the cook may put in some seaweed in the form of *wakame*. Slices of chopped vegetables may be added. The bowl is usually served with a lid on it to keep the soup warm. This nourishing bowl of soup is equivalent to a Westerner's morning bacon and eggs.

Misoshiru is actually similar in function to a bowl of porridge, offering low-Calorie warmth and a lot of nourishment. *Misoshiru* has a distinctive mellow-pungent flavor, hard to get accustomed to but quite pleasant when you do.

After the soup comes the traditional *o-kazu*, which means side dish or relish and often includes a portion of protein. The protein can be a slice of fish, a piece of chicken, a chunk of *tofu*, or possibly an egg or part of an egg. None of these "pieces" is very large.

A JEWEL IN A SETTING

In the middle of the breakfast, more or less like a jewel in a setting, lies the *pièce de résistance*—the *umeboshi*, a tiny red plum pickled for eating. It is, in a sense, "nature's own mouthwash"—just one taste has the ability to straighten out your hair and send lightning flashes through your body. The plum is so sour that it *has* to be pickled to be eaten.

Selections of pickled vegetables also adorn most Japanese breakfast tables, although they are not essentially a dish in themselves but simple ornamentations.

Of course, the meal ends with a cup of good warm green tea.

As you can see, the main parts of the meal are the porridgelike soup and the bowl of rice with seaweed enhancement. These are the essentials that give the breakfast its food value. Much of the rest is embellishment on the main dishes.

A typical American meal of cereal, orange juice, and tea or coffee is surprisingly similar to a Japanese breakfast in caloric content and in nutritional value. In the suggested menus in Chapter 12, a typical American breakfast can always be substituted for the Japanese meal; it's hard to get used to thick soup and a heaping bowl of rice just after rolling out of bed!

Nevertheless, if you feel adventurous, you should try a Japanese meal in its entirety to see how it goes down. For breakfast you'll have trouble locating *umeboshi,* but that's not an essential. It's good to note that the pickled vegetables are not like Western pickled vegetables—sweet and dill. The Japanese pickle their vegetables in white-rice vinegar, with other condiments to flavor them. The pickling is not quite so tart and sharp as ours.

Let's move on to a typical lunch that might be served in a Japanese home.

THE LEFTOVERS FROM DINNER: A TYPICAL LUNCH

Most lunches are made up of leftovers from other meals— from dinner the night before, or possibly from breakfast. The bowl of rice becomes the center of the lunch meal. It may be rice in the pot left over from breakfast. Or a bowl of noodles can be substituted for rice. In modern Japan over four billion packages of dried instant noodles are sold each year!

In addition to the bowl of rice, there is usually a cup of clear broth soup—*suimono*—decorated or embellished with garnishes of all kinds.

To flavor the rice or noodles, the cook may add a few slices of raw fish, or *sashimi*.

In addition, the rice may be flavored by *furikake*, which is a type of seasoning combining a number of different flavorings and foodstuffs: *katsuobushi* (dried bonito), seaweeds, sesame seeds, egg, fish, tea, toasted *nori* (laver), and other flavorings. This condiment is sprinkled on the rice from a bottle with a perforated top. The meal may also consist of pieces of fried shrimp left over from the night before. Then there are always pickled vegetables to eat. And a cup of green tea to top it all off.

There are any number of variations on certain lunch dishes. Although rice is supposed to be eaten plain or not at all, there are occasions when certain foodstuffs can be poured over it, especially tea. One type of rice lunch is called *chazuke*, which means "soaked in tea." You pour a cup of tea over your rice and then drink the mixture, ending the meal with another cup of tea. This is a practice that is enjoyed at home, but not in public.

Many cooks have favorite recipes for *chazuke* that include slices of *sashimi*, slivers of salted fish, and *nori*, *katsuobushi*, or pickles of various kinds. Once these ingredients have been placed on or next to the rice, the tea is poured over the rice, which then is eaten with chopsticks.

A subvariation consists of substituting *dashi*, the soup stock of bonito and kelp, for the tea, and pouring *that* over the rice.

Noodles (*udon*, *soba*, *somen*, and so on) play an important role in the Japanese lunch. A large bowl of piping-hot noodles in winter and a basket of ice-cold noodles in summer are still the most popular lunches you can serve in Japan.

Hot noodles are usually prepared with seasoned *dashi* and topped with a large portion of garnish—chicken, egg, fried shrimp (*tempura*), fried bean curd (*abura-age*), fishcake (*kamaboko*), and so on—mixed with vegetables. In summer, cold noodles are often served with a small bowl of *tsuke-dashi* (cold seasoned *dashi*), with garnishes on the side. You pick up the noodles with a pair of chopsticks and dip them in the *tsuke-dashi* just before eating.

Shichimi-togarashi (seven-flavored spice), *wasabi* (Japanese horseradish), grated ginger, chopped scallion, and crumbed *nori* are often served with noodles to whet the appetite.

THE MAIN MEAL IN JAPAN: DINNER

Dinner usually consists of a number of dishes along with the traditional rice and soup.

Before looking at the most important meal in detail, let's discuss some basic principles of food preparation in Japan.

NOTE: It is impossible to understand today's traditional Japanese cuisine without comparing and contrasting it with a style of cooking called *shojin ryori*. *Shojin ryori* is also known as temple cooking.

COLOR AND TASTE IN JAPANESE MENUS

The Japanese pay a great deal of attention to color in their food servings. It has already been explained that there is a definite art in setting a Japanese table so as to whet the appetite of the diner to the utmost.

This preoccupation with color goes back many centuries to *shojin ryori* (*shojin* cooking). *Shojin* cuisine is prepared mainly in Zen Buddhist temples. Buddha stressed the virtuosity of vegetables; the *shojin* diet consisted only of vegetables, with, of course, seaweed quite properly considered as a vegetable.

One of the most important aspects of *shojin* cuisine was its emphasis on three principal elements in eating: taste variation, cooking variation, and color variation.

THE SIX TASTE VARIATIONS

In *shojin* cooking the chef tries to arrange the six basic taste variations so that the food will be balanced in lightness and softness, in cleanliness and freshness, and in precision and care.

The six basic tastes are:

bitter
sweet
salty
sour
hot
"delicate"

Balancing these taste sensations is a difficult and almost impossible chore for the busy cook today, but it is a consideration that still enters into Japanese cooking—and can enter into yours.

THE FIVE METHODS OF COOKING

Although there are more than five different methods of cooking practiced in Japan, the *shojin* chef uses only five:

boiling
grilling
deep frying
steaming
raw

Actually, the above methods do comprise all the types discussed in Chapter 9.

THE FIVE COLORS OF CUISINE

It is the *shojin* concept of the five colors of food that is the most interesting. The *shojin* cook tries to balance five basic colors in every meal if possible:

> green
> yellow
> red
> white
> black

NOTE: In foodstuffs a deep purple is considered black by the *shojin* cook. Eggplant is black. So is *kombu* (seaweed).

HOW TO THINK SMALL IN A BIG WAY

There are many different ways to serve a dinner in the Japanese fashion. In Japan dinner is the main meal just as it is in the United States.

Nevertheless, in spite of many similarities, there are fundamental differences between Japanese and American cuisine. One of the most important differences is the size of a moderate serving.

A glance at a typical Japanese menu and a study of what goes into a dinner will produce almost instant misunderstanding on the part of the American reader. What we would call the "main dish" might include some poultry items—pieces of chicken breast, for example. A side dish of salad might include shrimp. Another side dish might include pieces of beef.

That represents three different types of animal: poultry, shellfish, and beef! Instantly, you might assume this means a good healthy serving of chicken breast, the same of shrimp, and the same of beef.

33

And assuming the average American serving of meat of any kind is about 6 ounces or maybe even 8 ounces—look at any cookbook—that would make a pound and a half of meat!

Nothing could be further from the truth. You have to rethink your values. The Japanese do not—repeat, *do not*—eat anywhere near the amount of meat Americans do.

Typically, the *entire* nonvegetable portion of a typical Japanese meal would include not much more than 4 ounces of animal protein—chicken breast, shrimp, *and* beef—in all. In some households, in fact, the total amount of nonvegetable foodstuffs for the dinner described above might be as low as 2 ounces.

The picture of a typical Japanese meal is tiny portions of many different types of foodstuffs—put together in various colors, shapes, and designs.

LOOK WHAT'S COMING FOR DINNER

Let's translate this basic idea—great variety in food selection, small amounts of each dish—by looking at a typical Japanese dinner.

The meal would have a menu like this:

rice
soup
main dish
vegetable in season
seafood in season
pickled vegetables
fruit
tea

That's eight items!
But only one dish—what serves as the main dish but

which is not specified in the list above—is large. It might be *sukiyaki,* to take one of the best-known Japanese dishes. Some of the "vegetables in season" would be included in the *sukiyaki* dish. The "seafood in season" might be included in some kind of condiment or appetizer, tiny and quickly eaten. The pickled vegetables might be one very small piece of cabbage. The fruit for dessert might be only a slice of peach.

Even Japanese recipe books can be deceiving to the American cook. Most of the recipes concentrate only on a so-called main-course dish. But these dishes are grouped in such a way that the unwary American cook might prepare two or three main courses for *one* dinner!

It's not that some Japanese who are rich and want to eat like Diamond Jim Brady might *not* serve themselves two main courses for dinner. It's that the average Japanese does not eat quite so lavishly. Japan is a country that resists conspicuous consumption.

SEVEN MENUS FEATURING JAPANESE DISHES

In the following section, there are seven menus containing Japanese and Japanese-style dishes for you to look at. Several of the items in each menu are included in the recipe section at the back of the book in Chapter 10. The recipes will tell you how to cook the dish and (when necessary) how to serve it. Items marked with an asterisk are in the recipe section.

You should realize that the inclusion of chicken, seafood, and beef in one meal does *not* mean a heaping plate of each, but only a small amount of one and probably only a nibble of the other two.

Seven Menus Featuring Japanese Dishes

Menu 1

rice
clear soup with chicken*
tempura (featuring shrimp)* with *tempura* dip*
grated *daikon* (radish) and gingerroot as condiments*
cucumber and sesame-seed salad*
fruit
tea

NOTE: *Tempura* means "deep-fried shrimp" in America, but the word originally simply meant "deep-fried food." Deep frying was introduced to the Japanese by Portuguese seamen centuries ago. Other foodstuffs can be deep-fried for *tempura* variations.

Menu 2

rice
clear soup* with shredded pork and vegetables (carrots, Chinese mushrooms, scallions, or bamboo shoots)
yakitori (featuring chicken)*
green beans with ginger*
fruit
tea

NOTE: The main course, *yakitori,* means chicken grilled on skewers over a charcoal fire. But you can substitute beef or seafood in this menu.

Menu 3

rice

miso soup* with *tofu* and seaweed

teriyaki (featuring salmon)*

spinach with lemon sauce*

fruit

tea

NOTE: The main course is *teriyaki*, literally "shining broil," but generally meaning broiled marinated seafood, poultry, or meat. Seafood or poultry can be substituted at any time to vary the main dish. See the recipe in Chapter 10.

Menu 4

sushi cucumber bars*

shabu-shabu (featuring beef)*

ponzu dipping sauce*

fruit

tea or *sake*

NOTE: This is a one-pot meal, featuring food cooked at the table by the diners themselves. See discussion in Chapter 9.

Menu 5

hiya-yakko (cold *tofu* dish)*

rice

egg-drop soup*

shioyaki (featuring white-meat fish)*

carrot *namasu*ter*

whole simmered okra pods*
fruit
tea

NOTE: *Shioyaki* (cooking by salt-broiling) can feature any kind of fish. The recipe in Chapter 10 is for freshwater trout. Whitefish or mackerel can be substituted with ease.

Menu 6

rice
clear soup* with clams and lime peel
broiled chicken livers*
chawanmushi (featuring egg)*
spinach *sunomono**
fruit
tea

NOTE: *Chawanmushi* is a steamed custardlike dish with some fish and vegetables in it. It is, of course, not sweet but slightly salty. The terms *sunomono* and *namasu* both refer to what a Westerner might call a salad. However, there is a subtle difference. *Namasu* usually refers to vegetables and some seafood marinated in vinegared sauce. *Sunomono* usually refers to vegetables and seafood mixed with a vinegared sauce just before serving.

Menu 7

rice
prawn and cucumber soup*
umani (vegetables and chicken)*
Chinese cabbage in vinegar*

fruit

tea

NOTE: The word *umani* means "deliciously cooked," and refers to vegetables, meat, poultry, fish, or dried food cooked in *dashi* and seasoned lightly with *sake,* soy sauce, salt, and *mirin* (rice wine used for cooking) until the liquid is practically all absorbed.

PART TWO:

Magic Lightweight Foods

Chapter 4

RICE: THE HONORABLE FOOD

In Japan no food is respected more than rice. Noodles, served as a substitute for rice, are not esteemed in the same way. Although these two foods are the mainstays of the Japanese diet, rice has the edge in prestige and clout. Proof lies in the fact that the word *gohan,* which is the word for a rice meal, also means "meal." (Actually, the word for rice is *kome,* but that refers to uncooked rice.)

During the spring and autumn months, the Japanese celebrate Inari, the rice god, and Ukemochi-no-kami, the food goddess. There are dozens of different ways of serving rice—but plain boiled rice is the staple of the Japanese table.

It all started several centuries before Christ when the cultivation of rice was brought to Japan from the Chinese mainland. *Kojiki,* the oldest existing document on Japanese history, written in 720 A.D., suggests that rice was respected at that time more than any other grain. There are several reasons for its ancient and continued popularity. First, the crop yield from a unit of land is better than most other grains. Second, the retention of the edible part of the grain is greater than other crops. Third, rice is easily stored. Fourth, it is easier to cook than most other grains. And fifth, repeated consumption of rice does not adversely affect the palate.

One can estimate that an average Japanese grown-up eats about two hundred pounds of rice each year, from the data compiled by the Ministry of Agriculture and Forestry of Japan. By comparison, the average American consumes nine pounds of rice. It is an inexpensive foodstuff, far cheaper than potatoes and similar vegetables.

THE EXCEPTIONAL QUALITIES OF RICE

Rice does not have a large quantity of protein; however, what it lacks in quantity it makes up for in protein *quality*. Rice has most of the essential amino acids in the proper proportion. Essential amino acids are those that cannot be synthesized in the body and yet are essential for body composition and function. In order to enable the body to use dietary protein effectively for these purposes, the protein must contain all the essential amino acids in the proper proportion.

Rice is also a good source of digestible complex carbohydrates. Its digestibility depends on the degree of polishing, with the most polished rice being the most digestible.

Rice's most important quality is its ability to provide for "protein sparing." This is a term nutritionists use to describe the ability of a foodstuff to permit someone to cut down safely on the portions of meat he or she needs for a balanced diet.

For example, rice will supply the eater with enough energy (contained in its carbohydrates) that the protein from any meat consumed can be used for what it does best: build and repair body cells. Rice thus allows the dieter to eat less meat and avoid the intake of needless fat and cholesterol.

To elaborate on this point a bit, there is one drawback to certain proteins supplied by animals and vegetables: They are only "partially complete" proteins. For example, the protein in some fish contains relatively little methionine—one of the essential amino acids mentioned above. Proteins from vegetables supply only small amounts of one or another of the essential amino acids—lysine, methionine, or tryptophan.

One vegetable alone cannot supply the full advantage of protein; only a part of that vegetable's total protein can be used. However, by combining two or more vegetable proteins—say, rice protein and soybean protein, pea protein and sesame-seed protein—a complementary protein is achieved. That means that in a varied vegetable diet you can create a complete protein.

The Japanese usually serve rice with other protein-containing foods like the soybean itself, or with derivatives of soybeans, like *tofu* (bean curd) or *miso* (bean paste). Rice and *tofu* form a complete protein and together become an effective nutrient.

WHY RICE IS GOOD FOR YOU

Now, let's take a close look at the nutritional composition of rice. Different kinds of rice have different makeups, but the disposition of nutrients is about the same for all types.

- One cup of uncooked long-grain white rice has a caloric count of about 672. The breakdown of the principal nutrients providing that caloric count is: 13.7 grams of protein, 150.0 grams of carbohydrate, 0.6 gram of fat.
- One cup of cooked white rice has a caloric count of about 186 Calories: 3.7 grams of protein, 40.4 grams of carbohydrate, 0.2 gram of fat.
- As for uncooked brown rice, one cup pro-

vides 666 Calories: 13.9 grams of protein,
141.5 grams of carbohydrate, and 3.5 grams
of fat.

It is obvious that the carbohydrate content of rice is very high. And automatically you think, "bad." There is a very good reason for this reaction. You have been brainwashed, to a degree, about the carbohydrate content of foods. Nutritionists have always reminded people on diets that candy, cookies, cakes, and pies—all of which are filled with carbohydrates—cause overweight.

CARBOHYDRATES *ARE* GOOD FOR YOU!

In a way, the common carbohydrate has really been given a bad name through the years. In some popular diets, the carbohydrate count is kept deliberately low in order to cause the dieter to lose weight.

There are two basic types of carbohydrates—starches (called complex carbohydrates) and sugars (called simple carbohydrates). There are also two kinds of each type: "natural" carbohydrates, found in nature, and "refined" or "processed" carbohydrates, like granulated sugar, extracted from natural sources and used as additives in food preparation.

In natural foodstuffs, starches and sugars are mixed with a wide variety of essential nutrients, with a satisfactory ratio of nutrients to Calories. When refined carbohydrates are used as additives in rich pastries, the resultant Calories are known as "empty Calories."

A glance at the nutritional information on a package of granulated pure cane sugar will tell you why: One level teaspoon of processed sugar contains 5 grams of carbohydrates (19 Calories)—but 0.0 grams of protein and 0.0 grams of fat.

In spite of the fact that most types of rice contain large amounts of carbohydrates, they also provide essential protein and, at the same time, little or no fat. Brown rice has more fat in it than white rice, but that amount is negligible compared with the ratio between protein and fat in animal meat.

Rice is a starchy food, like most other grains. Starch absorbs a lot of water, increasing the bulk of the rice a great deal when it is cooked. Thus it can fulfill both your physical and psychological needs for food. When you finish a bowl of rice, you know that you've eaten something. It sticks to your ribs, so to speak. At least temporarily.

Rice is indeed, as the Japanese discovered thousands of years ago, a miracle food—one that is usually served at every traditional Japanese meal and is eaten from beginning to end as a supplement to all the rest of the dishes.

WHAT THE MIRACLE FOOD DOES FOR YOU

As for energy, the Rice Council of America says that ½ cup of rice produces enough body energy to allow you to walk 3 miles an hour for thirty-five minutes and 8 seconds.

Rice has the capacity of being digested rapidly, in only one hour. Other foodstuffs take much longer. Rice is ideal for people on low-sodium and low-fat diets; it contains only traces of sodium and fat, and it has absolutely no cholesterol.

Most rice is enriched with iron, thiamine, and niacin. Brown rice is naturally rich in iron, thiamine, and niacin as well as vitamin E, and it is not enriched. Brown rice takes longer to cook because of the high ether and oil content of its bran layer.

Brown rice expands during cooking. The bran coating "explodes" and the bran adheres to the rice grain, forming a tender, firm texture. The bran layer is as tender as the inside grain. Brown rice tastes different from white rice; it has a more nutlike flavor.

NOTE: Brown rice should not be confused with wild rice, which is not even in the same family. Wild rice usually goes well with chicken and turkey, with pheasant and quail, and with any delicately flavored food like oysters and mushrooms. However, it is quite expensive in comparison with white rice and brown rice.

To ensure getting all the nutritional value from rice, it must be prepared and cooked properly. Here's the way to do it in the Japanese fashion:

> You'll need between 1 and 2 cups of water to cook a cup of polished rice. The amount of water varies with the kind of rice used. The Japanese like to use about 20 percent more water than rice, using Japanese-variety rice. Every cook must experiment to find the proper balance between water and rice; it all depends on your personal taste. Once you have determined the proper ratio of water to rice, wash the rice in many changes of water until it is clean, or no longer cloudy. Drain the rice and place in a 1-quart covered saucepan. Add water. Bring the rice to a boil, then reduce the heat, and cover pan, letting it simmer for about 15 minutes.
>
> For brown rice, use from 1 to 2½ cups of water for every cup. Boil the rice, stir, and cover pan. Then let it simmer for 45 to 55 minutes. Brown rice will be as tender as regular rice only when it has been fully cooked.

THE DIFFERENT FACES OF RICE

No meal in Japan, for the rich or for the poor, is complete without rice. For the Japanese it is like meat and potatoes are for Westerners. Every meal—breakfast, lunch, and dinner—contains a bowl of hot or cold rice.

Rice is most often served along with any other course of a meal, except when *sake* is drunk. However, once the *sake* is gone, a rice course winds up the meal.

Sometimes rice is served with fish, meat, or vegetables, which are either mixed with the rice or placed on top of it. This type of serving is known as *meshimono,* or "rice foods." Plain steamed rice however rates as the general favorite among the Japanese.

Steamed rice has a delicate and somewhat bland taste, particularly to Westerners. That blandness is delicately accented with other food flavors. However, unless the rice is properly cooked, it is likely to be sticky and flavorless. Correct preparation is extremely important.

In a Japanese kitchen, a heavy, covered cooking pot called a *kama* was traditionally used for rice. The *kama* was placed on a *kamado,* a type of stove, and watched during cooking. Electric pots designed especially to cook rice, called "electric rice cookers," are now used widely.

Any heavy, thick-bottomed pan with a tight-fitting lid can be used to cook rice. If a pressure cooker is the only implement available, it too can be utilized, as long as the amount of water is reduced. The rice must be boiled under pressure for about 7 minutes and kept under pressure for another 10 minutes after the heat is turned off.

HOW TO PERK UP A BOWL OF RICE

Don't get the idea that there is no way to add to the bland flavor of rice. There is. It is permissible—in fact, in some instances preferable—to garnish rice with various kinds of foodstuffs.

In *shojin* cooking, rice dishes are varied each season with garnishes and decorations that cause them to be called "color rice" dishes:

- During the winter, you can cook dried soybeans with rice; or you can add fresh ginger, thinly sliced and cut into "needle" pieces, to the top of rice.
- During the spring, you can add boiled green peas to rice; or you can add *okara,* the residue left when boiled soybeans have been ground and strained for making *tofu.*
- During the summer, you can sprinkle perilla leaves or mint leaves on cooked rice; or you can add chestnuts during the cooking.
- During the fall, you can add and cook ginkgo nuts, cubed sweet potato, or mushroom bits with rice.
- For a general, all-season garnish, you can always add *azuki* beans and cook together with rice.

Not only do these additions help the flavor of the rice—it is quite a tasteless grain if cooked and eaten without enhancement—but they also help to brighten up the glaring whiteness of the rice dish itself with a bit of welcome color.

THE DIFFERENT GRADES OF RICE

Rice comes in all grades:

- In the best grade, all the grains are of uniform size and shape. Each possesses a dull, pearly luster.

- In the medium and poor grades, the grains are of different sizes and shapes.
- The cook must use different amounts of water with each grade of rice. With the best grade, less water; with the poorest, more. The proportion of water to rice is only slightly more than almost double.
- One cup of uncooked rice produces about 4 cups of cooked rice.
- Cup for cup, rice absorbs anywhere between its own volume of water to twice its volume.

Rice is also the base of a Japanese vinegar called *su*. *Su*, a clear and amber-colored liquid with a sweet, aromatic quality much different from the cider (apple) vinegar Americans are used to, is made from white rice and malted rice, from *sake*, or from the lees of *sake*. If a Japanese rice vinegar is not available for a recipe, you can always substitute distilled cider vinegar.

Rice can also be used to make various types of wafers. One of the most popular is called *senbei*, a thin cracker prepared from rice flour and egg. Sesame seeds, laver seaweed, soy sauce, and other ingredients can also be added. These wafers are eaten as snacks between meals.

Mochi, a sticky rice cake, eaten during the New Year's holiday, is made from glutinous rice. Steamed rice is patted until it becomes the consistency of smooth, sticky paste. It is then formed into small disks or other shapes and dried. The pieces are often toasted and served with soy sauce and seaweed, or put into a type of soup. This dish is called *zoni*.

SAKE AND MIRIN

Rice is used as the base of *sake*, the Japanese national alcoholic drink. *Sake* has an alcoholic content of about 17 percent, the same as that of a strong European wine. It is prepared as follows:

- First the rice is steamed and malted with a mold spore.
- Once this mash is prepared, it is mixed with water and a yeast culture to hasten fermentation.
- After a month, this fermented mixture is filtered and bottled.
- Both the kind of rice and the quality of the water used in the wine have a great deal to do with the quality of the final product.

A sweet, less strong wine known as *mirin* is also used for cooking. This cooking wine is often mixed with soy sauce in the recipes. If no *sake* is available, a very dry sherry, slightly diluted with water, can be substituted without losing the entire flavor. White Port or cream sherry can be used as substitutes for *mirin*.

Chapter 5

VEGETABLES: BUDDHA'S INSPIRATION

Although the Japanese were not always vegetarians and were introduced to that integral part of their diet by Buddhist monks—in particular the Zen Buddhists, as mentioned in Chapter 3—they became fascinated with the variety and versatility of vegetables during the following centuries, and today include them in a greater portion of their daily diet than almost any other people.

In the Japanese menu, there is little distinction between salads and vegetables. A vegetable that might be cooked in America may be served uncooked and at room temperature in Japan. Nevertheless, whether it is used cooked as a vegetable or uncooked as a salad, vegetables generally form part of a meal and occupy as important a position as fish, poultry, meat, or soup and rice.

The Japanese make their vegetable dishes both simple and complex. Their aim is to produce a fresh, natural food. Most important to the American borrowing the Japanese philosophy of cuisine, the Japanese penchant for using vegetables heavily in the daily diet helps cut down total caloric intake—particularly from saturated fats—in a dramatic fashion.

For example, an average serving of a typical boiled vegetable, like bean sprouts, cabbage, celery, cucumber, mushrooms, spinach, or Swiss chard, contains only 1 to 15 Calories, and an average serving of bamboo shoots, carrots, eggplant, fennel, scallions, and turnips contains only 16 to 25 Calories. Even starchy vegetables like lima beans and peas contain only around 50 Calories.

FAT IN THE TYPICAL JAPANESE DIET

Because of the predominance of vegetables and fish in the Japanese diet, one can easily hold down caloric intake from fat to less than 10 percent by eating traditional Japanese menus. Most of that fat is not from animal sources either, but "good" fat—polyunsaturated fat from vegetable sources. Only 3 percent of the total caloric intake of a Japanese diet comes from saturated fat.

Dr. Ancel Keys and his staff at the University of Minnesota found that as a result of their diet, the Japanese had very low cholesterol levels, and the death rate from coronary-artery disease in Japan was only 20 per 10,000, as opposed to 185 per 10,000 in the United States!

Another study determined that the low-fat diet of the Japanese also tends to control two types of cancer—cancer of the colon and cancer of the breast (the leading cancer killer of American women). These diseases have been found to be uncommon among the Japanese people, largely, it is thought, because of their low-fat diet.

When the Japanese emigrate to the United States and change their diet to conform to American custom, they tend to risk developing these diseases. Apparently, it is the high ratio of vegetables to meat in the Japanese diet that minimizes the occurrence of these types of cancer. As for breast cancer, there is five to ten times as much in the United States with its high-fat diet as in Japan with its low-fat diet.

In addition to their low caloric content—particularly in fats—many of these vegetables contain an active ingredient that has become most important in establishing weight control for diet-conscious people. That active ingredient is fiber. Not only does a high-fiber food provide nutritional values, but it tends to fill up the stomach, leaving the eater satisfied and less hungry for more food, as already mentioned in the discussion on rice in the preceding chapter.

Many vegetables in favorite Japanese dishes have a high-fiber content, including string beans, turnips, cabbage, Chinese cabbage, carrots, *daikon,* or white radish, and cucumbers.

As for vitamins, dark green and deep yellow vegetables are good sources of vitamin A; this group includes spinach, carrots, yams, and other vegetables. Most dried legumes, like peas, navy beans, and soybeans, provide copious amounts of protein along with the B vitamins, iron, and other important nutrients.

Nutritionists point out that it is advisable to eat three different kinds of vegetables daily: a dark green vegetable, a starchy vegetable, and any third type of vegetable. The dark green vegetable might be beet greens or spinach or string beans; the starchy vegetable might be lima beans; the third vegetable might be eggplant.

The Japanese have always used such combinations, not only in vegetable dishes but in salads as well.

An analysis of favorite Japanese vegetables from the standpoint of caloric content, high fiber content, vitamin content, and nutritional values in general shows that from the beginning, the traditional Japanese meal has always afforded excellent balance between these elements and provided effective control over weight gain.

THE SCARCITY OF DAIRY PRODUCTS

One basic point to remember in studying Japanese cuisine is that traditional dishes never included dairy products like butter, cream, or cheese. Vegetables have always been prepared without butter (a heavy source of saturated fat), but with salt, soy sauce, *mirin,* vinegar, sesame seeds, mustard, *tofu,* or *miso* (about which more later) in certain combinations. Japanese cooking oils are made from vegetable oils rather than from animal fats.

Note the lack of dairy products with their heavy concentration of saturated fat and cholesterol in the Japanese diet. It is the addition of saturated fat and cholesterol in the preparation of vegetables that Americans should avoid. The traditional Japanese diet bypasses this problem.

One of the key differences between typical Japanese vegetables and American vegetables is the Japanese inclusion of seaweed in its many forms. Not only is seaweed eaten as a vegetable, but it is used to form the basis of various kinds of dishes. For example, agar-agar, a jelling agent made from *tengusa,* or red seaweed, is used in many Japanese sweets and dishes. Laver, another kind of seaweed, is an important seasoning and garnish. *Kombu,* still another type, is also present in *dashi,* the basic stock for soups and other dishes. (Seaweed is covered later on in Chapter 7.)

A GUIDE TO TYPICAL JAPANESE VEGETABLES

What follows is a selected list of favorite Japanese vegetables. Because many of them are not available everywhere in the United States, and because many are used in the recipes at the back of this book, certain substitutes that can be used for the more esoteric vegetables have been indicated.

MAGIC LIGHTWEIGHT FOODS

Azuki Beans

These dried red beans are usually served with a sweetener, like sugar and/or honey. The *azuki* bean is actually a health-food delicacy and can sometimes be obtained in health-food stores in America. It appears in a bean jam called *an*, and in a jellylike sweet called *yokan*. The bean has a high fiber content. One serving (75 grams) of a half-cup of *azuki* beans, boiled in water, no sugar added, provides about 108 Calories in the following nutritional breakdown: 6.7 grams of protein, 16.8 grams of carbohydrate, and 0.8 gram of fat. This serving also contains 1.4 grams of fiber. Any small red bean may be substituted for the *azuki* bean.

Bamboo Shoots

Although bamboo, called *takenoko*, is simply a huge species of grass, the underground shoots can be used for food. Bamboo shoots should be peeled and then boiled before being incorporated into any dish. They have a nutty flavor. Cooked with meat, such as chicken, the shoots give the meat an added flavor. Shoots are a low-Calorie food, high in fiber.

Bean Sprouts

Called *moyashi* by the Japanese, bean sprouts are actually one of the most popular vegetables in China, where they have been used for over three thousand years. A half-cup of bean sprouts, about a normal serving, provides around 11 Calories: 1.2 grams of protein, 1.9 grams of carbohydrate, and only a trace of fat. It is a fairly high-fiber food, and contains a large amount of vitamin C (6 milligrams per serving).

Black Beans

Kuromame is a legume with a highly distinctive look. It has a creamy flesh and a strong, meaty flavor. Usually sold as a dried bean, it is cooked to make sweet beans—one of the typical Japanese New Year dishes. A half-cup of black beans provides 339 Calories: 28.5 grams of protein, 15.5 grams of carbohydrate, and 15.4 grams of fat. The beans have a high fiber content.

Burdock Root

Gobo is a skinny, woody root that must be soaked in vinegared water before preparation to prevent discoloration. Then it is often boiled and pounded with a wooden mallet before serving, or it is simmered in a seasoned stock for some time. It is a fairly rare item in the United States.

Carrots

Called *ninjin,* the carrot is one of the world's most important root vegetables, and has been cultivated for two thousand to three thousand years. The carrot is rich in vitamins, particularly vitamin A, and contains more natural sugar than any other vegetable except the beet. A 2-ounce serving provides about 24 Calories: 0.7 gram of protein, 4.7 grams of carbohydrate, and 0.1 gram of fat. It is a high-fiber vegetable (0.8 gram of fiber per 2-ounce serving).

Chinese Cabbage

Called *hakusai,* this "Chinese" cabbage is also known in America as Napa cabbage and celery cabbage. It is shaped differently from the more familiar Western cabbage, the head being as long as 16 inches. You can use Chinese cabbage raw for salads and for pickling; you can also use it as a dish by itself or in soup. If *hakusai* is not available, you can substitute almost any variety of ordinary cabbage or endive. A 4-ounce serving provides 14 Calories: 1.2 grams of protein, 2.4 grams of carbohydrate, and 0.1 gram of fat. It also has a high fiber content.

Coltsfoot

Fuki is a rhubarblike plant, with a long, green, hollow stalk. It must first be parboiled in salted water then destringed. It tastes remarkably like celery. If you do not find coltsfoot in the stores, you can substitute plain celery. Three stalks of celery weighing a little less than 2 ounces provide 8 Calories: 0.4 gram of protein, 2 grams of carbohydrate, and 0.1 gram of fat. It is a fibrous vegetable.

Crown Daisy

Shungiku, also known as the garland chrysanthemum, is a green vegetable grown for Japanese cookery. The daisy leaves can be eaten parboiled and can be flavored to taste. Also called "chop-suey greens," the crown daisy is a popular ingredient in *sukiyaki* and other dishes. It can be cooked by itself with soy sauce. You can always substitute dandelion leaves, spinach, chard, or mustard greens for the crown daisy, although the perfume and flavor, which are its most important aspects, will be lacking. This type of vegetable is a low-Calorie food. One 4-ounce serving of dandelion leaves, for example, provides about 40 Calories: 2.5 grams of protein, 5.7 grams of carbohydrate, and about 0.5 gram of fat. It is high in fiber content (1.5 grams per 4-ounce serving).

Eggplant

Nasubi has the same deep purple color as the American eggplant but is smaller and rounder. The skin is very tender. If *nasubi* is not available, you can substitute American eggplant. A 4-ounce serving provides about 30 Calories: 1.4 grams of protein, 5.5 grams of carbohydrate, and 0.2 gram of fat.

Gingerroot

Called *shoga,* gingerroot is probably one of the most widely used condiments in Japan. The rhizomes are usually grated, cut into needles or thin slices, and served in many different ways. Ginger slices, pickled in white vinegar, are called *gari* and are used as a condiment with *sushi.*

Ginkgo Nuts

The seeds of the female ginkgo, or maidenhair, tree are called *ginnan* by the Japanese. They can be steamed, skewered, grilled, deep-fried, or prepared for a separate dish. The ginkgo nut served roasted is a condiment. The fruit resembles a small greenish-yellow plum; it is the nut inside that is eaten.

Japanese Cucumber

Kyuri is crisper, narrower, smaller, and less watery than the American or European cucumber. It can be used in salads and vegetable dishes of all kinds. One cucumber of normal size provides about 38 Calories: 2.3 grams of protein, 7.1 grams of carbohydrate, and 0.1 gram of fat. A normal serving of 6 slices of cucumber, each slice about ⅛ inch in width, contains only 6 Calories!

MAGIC LIGHTWEIGHT FOODS

Long Onions

Negi are longer and thicker than scallions, but smaller than leeks. They have a surprisingly delicate flavor. You can slice and chop *negi* for any recipe requiring onions. If they are unavailable, you can substitute scallions. A 4-ounce serving contains about 28 Calories: 1.9 grams of protein, 4.3 grams of carbohydrate, and 0.2 gram of fat.

Lotus Root

Called *renkon* or *hasu,* the lotus root can be sliced, scalded in vinegared water, and used in salads. In some Japanese dishes, the lacy form of the sliced lotus root—created by the air spaces inside the flesh—can be used to make decorative shapes on the plate. It can be deep-fried or simmered.

Mountain Yam

Yama imo is bumpy on the outside and soft on the inside. It is a tuber like any other potato. It can be eaten raw with tuna or boiled rice and egg. You can boil it or fry it as a separate dish. One yam provides about 160 Calories: 3.3 grams of protein, 35 grams of carbohydrate, and 0.3 gram of fat.

Mushrooms

There is an almost endless variety of mushrooms popular with Japanese cooks and diners:

- *Enokitake* is a slender white mushroom. It is usually served raw or cooked in soups and other dishes.
- *Kikurage* is a thin dark mushroom, usually

sold dried. It is black and brittle and can be used in many different dishes.

• *Shiitake* is the most common mushroom and is sold dried. After soaking, it can be served in salads, it can be grilled, braised, simmered, or served as a dish in itself. It is said that *shiitake* lowers blood-cholesterol levels. It can be used in any *sukiyaki* and *tempura* recipe.

Any American mushroom can be substituted for a Japanese variety. The caloric content of mushrooms is low. A 4-ounce serving contains 32 Calories: 3 grams of protein, 4 grams of carbohydrate, and 0.3 gram of fat. The usual serving is probably less than 4 ounces unless prepared as a dish in itself.

Peas

Called *endo* by the Japanese, the fresh or frozen pea is a popular vegetable in Japanese dishes. A 4-ounce serving of boiled peas provides 80 Calories: 6 grams of protein, 11.3 grams of carbohydrate, and 0.4 gram of fat. Green peas have a high-fiber content.

Scallions

Called *wakegi,* these members of the onion family are usually chopped, diced, and minced as a garnish for salads, soups, sauces, and noodle recipes. A serving of about 3 ounces—probably more than you could eat at one sitting—provides about 27 Calories: 1.7 grams of protein, 5.5 grams of carbohydrate, and only a trace of fat.

Sesame Seeds

There are two kinds of *goma*, or sesame seeds: white and black. The black seeds are used for garnish. The white seeds are used in regular recipes. Try dry roasting the seeds to bring out the flavor. Sesame seeds can be used to flavor other foods, like rolls or bread or crackers. A teaspoon provides about 17 Calories: 0.6 gram of protein, 0.4 gram of carbohydrate, and 1.6 grams of fat. This quantity contains 36 milligrams of calcium.

Snow Peas

The *saya-endo* is a crisp, young pea pod, cultivated to be cooked and eaten whole, unlike the common-garden variety of pea. The snow pea is also called the sugar pea.

Soybeans

Called *daizu*, the dried soybean is available in stores throughout the United States. Fresh and immature soybeans are called *edamame*. The green pods can be boiled and served as a snack. A 4-ounce serving of boiled young soybeans from a can contains about 115 Calories: 10.1 grams of protein, 6.7 grams of carbohydrate, and 5.6 grams of highly unsaturated fat. If soybeans are not available, substitute lima beans or other similar legumes.

Squash

Kabocha is a squash very much like the pumpkin in taste and in shape, but it is smaller, with a brown or dark green skin rather than the familiar orange hue. If *kabocha* is not available, you can substitute either acorn squash or pumpkin. One half an acorn squash provides about 97 Calories:

3.3 grams of protein, 21.6 grams of carbohydrate, and 0.2 gram of fat. It is a high-fiber food.

Sweet Potato

Satsuma imo has a reddish outer skin and a golden interior. It is often sliced and served with *tempura* dishes. It can be sweet-simmered and eaten as a confectionary dish. A typical 4-ounce serving provides about 125 Calories: 3.3 grams of protein, 21.6 grams of carbohydrate, and 0.2 gram of fat (these values do not contain sugar). If unavailable, you can substitute yams.

Taro Potato

The field or country potato, called *sato imo,* is a member of the yam family. It has a dark brown, fuzzy skin and gray pulp inside. The taro potato can be boiled and served as a vegetable dish, or used in other recipes. If not available, small new potatoes can always be substituted.

Udo

Udo is a vegetable resembling fennel or spikenard, although it is grown out of the sunlight and is white and delicate in appearance. *Udo* is usually eaten raw, flavored only with vinegar dressing. It can be added to soup as a garnish. If *udo* is unobtainable, you can always substitute fennel, celery, or asparagus. It is a low-calorie food with a high fiber content. A serving of 6 spears of asparagus, for example, provides about 18 Calories: 2 grams of protein, 3 grams of carbohydrate, and just a trace of fat.

Wasabi

Wasabi, a member of the horseradish family, resembles celery root. It is the root itself that is edible; it must be peeled and grated. The Japanese use powdered *wasabi* in cooking the way Americans use mustard. *Wasabi* helps flavor *sushi* and *sashimi*. It can be added to soy sauce for a *sashimi* dipping sauce. If you cannot get *wasabi*, simply substitute white horseradish or spicy dried mustard.

White Radish

Called *daikon*, this large vegetable is completely edible. Very popular in Japan, it can be served raw, or it can be pickled or cooked in many ways. Grated, *daikon* is usually served with broiled fish or meat. Shredded, it commonly accompanies *sashimi* dishes. Softened and braised, *daikon* can be used as a vegetable dish on its own. A 4-ounce serving contains only 21 Calories: 1.0 gram of protein, 4 grams of carbohydrate, and a trace of unsaturated fat. If *daikon* is not available, you can substitute white turnip.

Chapter 6

THE ESSENTIALS OF JAPANESE COOKING

THE "MAGIC" OF THE SOYBEAN

Of all the vegetables mentioned, the most important is the soybean. This "magic" bean not only can grow on very poor soil, but it provides a most versatile food that can be served in some manner at almost every Japanese meal. Called the "meat of the field," the soybean is an invaluable source of protein.

Scientists have long said that if everyone on earth ate soybeans instead of meat, the planet could support sixteen billion people, rather than the current estimated four and a half billion. For example, an acre of soybeans can keep a moderately active man alive for 2,200 days; an acre of cattle graze would keep him for only seventy-five days.

Soy is the richest natural vegetable food known to man. The bean produces not only an edible vegetable, but oil, which can be used for cooking and as the basis for margarine. Mixed with cereal grains, the soybean can be fermented to produce soy sauce. The bean can be pulverized into a milk that approximates cow's milk.

This vegetable also forms the basis of *miso*, an ingredient made of soybeans and cereal grains fermented with water and salt for use in soups and sauces. Its residue, *tamari*, the liquid that rises to the top during fermentation, was probably the inspiration for soy sauce. *Moyashi*, the tender young sprouts of the soybean, are cultivated on indoor racks.

The vegetable needs only moisture and good drainage to grow and flourish. Within a few days, a cup of soybeans can produce three to four pounds of sprouts! Dried beans are ground, soaked in water, cooked and mashed, then sieved through a sheet of cloth to obtain soybean milk. The milk is coagulated with the aid of a natural coagulant to produce *tofu*, or bean curd, another staple of the Japanese diet. Steamed and fermented beans become *natto*, a condiment the Japanese all seem to love.

Shoyu

One of the principal condiments of the Japanese diet— *shoyu* (soy sauce)—is a direct descendant of the soybean. With its salty, slightly sweet, and meaty taste, it has spread from the Orient all over the world. The Orient uses *shoyu* as much as the West uses salt and pepper.

Soy sauce is made by first boiling the soybean until it is tender, then pounding it to a thin dust. Meanwhile, wheat or barley is grilled until dark brown, then crushed. The two ingredients—soy dust and crushed grain—are mixed together and put in a warm place, where malt seed is added. This substance, which is now a mash, is allowed to ferment. Salt is added and the mixture is left to mature for eighteen months. During these eighteen months, it is stirred and beaten occasionally.

At the end of the fermentation and maturation period, the mash that results is pressed through cloth, put into a tub, and left to settle. When the mash clears up, the liquid that is left is ready to be used as soy sauce, or *shoyu.*

Miso

Another multipurpose seasoning and foodstuff in Japanese cuisine is called *miso,* a paste made from fermented soybeans and other grains. After the soybeans are mixed with either rice malt or barley, they are combined with salt, water, and *Aspergillus oryzae* (a mold starter), and allowed to ferment. There are three main classifications of *miso:*

- *Aka:* Red to dark brown, this is a pungent type.
- *Chu:* Medium to golden, this is a mild type.
- *Shiro:* White to pale tan, this is a mellow type and slightly sweet to the taste.

The good news for dieters is that *miso* is composed primarily of oils that do not contain saturated fat or cholesterol. *Miso* can be eaten either as a condiment or as a relish; it can be used as a seasoning agent, a pickling agent, a soup or sauce base—somewhat like a bouillon cube—a soup or sauce thickener, a dressing or topping, or a spread or marinade.

Tofu

Another important derivative of the soybean is bean curd, called *tofu* by the Japanese. Because it is a source of high-quality protein, *tofu* has become a standard item in the health-food shops of America as well as in some supermarket chains. *Tofu* is rich also in important minerals and vitamins. It is free from cholesterol, low in saturated fat and calories, and easy to digest. These three facts are the principal reasons for its importance in a natural diet.

The nutritional composition of *tofu* largely depends on its water content. Chinese *tofu* is more concentrated than Japanese *momen-tofu*. The values cited here are those of Japanese *momen-tofu*. One 4-ounce serving contains 12 percent of the recommended daily allowance of protein, 17 percent of iron and calcium, 6 percent of thiamine, 2 percent of riboflavin. Its nutritional breakdown is as follows. One 4-ounce serving provides 86 Calories: 7.6 grams of protein, 1.0 gram of carbohydrate, 5.6 grams of unsaturated fat, 134 milligrams of calcium, and 1.6 milligrams of iron.

Tofu comes in a custardlike cake, often packaged in a plastic container. Once it is opened, it must be kept covered with water and refrigerated. A cooking ingredient, it is usually added to simple recipes for enhancing soups, salads, and omelets. In Japan there are many different forms of *tofu:*

- *Momen-tofu:* regular *tofu*
- *Kinugoshi-tofu:* a "silken" type
- Chinese-style *tofu:* a firm variety
- *Abura-age,* or *age:* deep-fried *tofu* puffs
- *Atsu-age,* or *nama-age:* deep-fried *tofu* cutlets, cakes, or cubes
- *Ganmo:* deep-fried *tofu* burgers
- *Yaki-dofu:* grilled *tofu.* (Note the substitution of "d" for "t" in the spelling.)
- *Koya-dofu:* freeze-dried *tofu*

Although not a magical ingredient, *tofu* is one of the key diet weapons in the Japanese arsenal of good health.

DASHI: THE SECRET OF JAPANESE FLAVOR

There is one more basic food element that is of primary importance not only in Japanese cooking, but in dieting as well. This is *dashi,* a basic soup and food stock essential to

Japanese cuisine. It is recognized by chefs as the "corner-stone of Japanese cooking."

Literally, *dashi* means stock, including chicken or vege-table broth or any other type. The Japanese, however, are reluctant to use this word for any stock except those utilized in Japanese cooking. If chicken broth is used for Japanese cooking, it is called "chicken *dashi*," otherwise, the term is "chicken stock."

The most widely used *dashi* is made from dried bonito flakes, called *katsuobushi,* and a dark, dried kelp called *kombu.* Note that this ingredient is not strictly a vegetable base but is mixed in with fish. *Dashi* can in fact be made from a number of other foodstuffs, including mushrooms, fresh fish, dried fish, seaweed only, chicken, and so on.

Dashi gives soup a definitely Oriental flavor. For typical Western tastes, it might seem a bit fishy when first sampled. It can always be diluted, or used sparingly until you become accustomed to it.

The recipes of the two most basic *dashi*—soup stock, called *ichiban dashi,* and food stock, called *niban dashi*—are given in Chapter 10.

AVAILABILITY OF THE FOUR ESSENTIALS

These four essentials—*shoyu* (soy sauce), *tofu* (bean curd), *miso* (soybean paste), and *dashi* (stock)—are the main ele-ments of Japanese cuisine. It is not difficult to find soy sauce in America, although the Japanese use a much milder form than is customary in the United States. *Tofu* and *miso* can be found in health-food stores and supermarkets in most parts of this country. *Dashi* ingredients are sometimes difficult to obtain. If you cannot find them, you can always substitute chicken broth for the *dashi.*

Chapter 7

SEAFOOD: THE PERFECT NOURISHMENT

Never forget that Japan is a country of four main islands and more than three thousand small ones. With little space on land to grow food or graze cattle, the Japanese for centuries have relied on the sea for a large proportion of their nutrition. Although the Japanese diet includes seafood and meat and poultry, it is seafood that is the mainstay.

Food from the sea includes not only fish and shellfish but seaweed as well. All three of these foodstuffs are used in the day-to-day diet of the average Japanese.

The variety of fish and shellfish in the waters surrounding the islands of Japan is astonishing. The Japanese believe in eating food from the sea in the same way they eat food from the earth—in the closest form to nature possible. In effect, a Japanese gourmet eats fresh fish in its raw state—*sushi* and *sashimi*—much as a European gourmet eats steak *tartare*.

Seafood is packed with nutritional food values, and the package contains a great deal of noncaloric elements that help in maintaining a good weight-conscious diet. A serving of fish prepared the Japanese way (more about that later) and apportioned in the Japanese way, with a helping limited at most to 4 ounces, and in many cases 2 ounces or less, may provide only around 100 Calories per serving.

Fish is also high in protein. For that reason, seafood in all its forms—fish, shellfish, and seaweed—can be an invaluable aid in maintaining proper weight.

FISH—SEAFOOD NUMBER 1

Fish, particularly saltwater fish, can be eaten raw, or it can be eaten cooked in several different ways. Freshwater fish, on the other hand, can be eaten raw only with a great deal of care because of the possible presence of parasites.

Here are a number of special favorites with the Japanese:

Albacore

A type of tuna, albacore is a particular favorite of the Tokyo *sushi* and *sashimi* addict. Albacore is peachy to rose in color, with soft flesh. The Japanese call this fish *shiro maguro.* A 3½-ounce serving of albacore contains 180 Calories: 23 grams of protein, no carbohydrate, and 9 grams of fat.

Barracuda

Kamasu is another favorite fish in Japan, but the Japanese prefer the smaller variety—about 8 inches long. The giant barracuda familiar to American fishermen is not a popular food in the islands.

Carp

Called *koi,* the carp, because of its long life and its ability to swim against the current, is a symbol of success in career, translated by the Japanese into a macho sign of masculine virtue. Carp is preferred raw in *sushi* and *sashimi* dishes. It is also served cooked, often with *miso*. This long-lived fish sometimes attains fifty years and weighs forty-four pounds. Highly esteemed, it has firm flesh, and bones that are easy to remove. However, the smaller variety is actually preferred. A 3½-ounce serving contains about 115 Calories: 18 grams of protein, no carbohydrate, and 4 grams of fat.

Cod

Most Japanese cod, or *tara*, is the Atlantic type of codfish. This is the world's greatest commercial fish, with its tender, edible white flesh. Cod is related to the haddock. When young, it is marketed as scrod. Cod, served in many different ways, is often used by the Japanese for fishcakes, *kamaboko* and *chikuwa*. A 3½-ounce serving provides about 78 Calories: 17.6 grams of protein, no carbohydrate, and 0.3 gram of fat.

Eel

Freshwater eel is called *unagi,* saltwater eel, *anago.* The Japanese prefer *unagi.* Both kinds, however, can be served. They are usually prepared with a light brushing of sweet sauce called *tare.* *Anago* (saltwater eel) is then served for *sushi.* Grilled *unagi* (freshwater eel) is commonly served as is and called *kabayaki;* or it can be placed on the top of piping-hot rice and called *unadon;* it is rarely served in *sushi.* A 2-ounce serving of smoked eel—the preparation most familiar to Americans—contains 188 Calories: 10.6 grams of protein, no carbohydrate, and 15.8 grams of fat.

Octopus

Tako, octopus, is one of the mollusks of the sea, and has eight tentacles. Because of its rather nonappetizing appearance, most Americans wouldn't dream of eating it. The Japanese, however, have relished its savor ever since prehistoric times. It is the tentacles that make a delicious dish. *Tako,* in the style most widely appreciated called *sudako,* is simple, chilled slices of salt-boiled tentacles garnished with vinegared soy sauce and grated ginger.

Squid

Ika, squid, varies in size from as small as 1 inch in diameter to many feet across. While not actually an octopus, the squid resembles the octopus and has similar tentacles. However, with the squid, the most appreciated part is the flesh and not the tentacles. *Ika's* chalky-white flesh can be eaten both raw and cooked. Dried, its flesh makes a delicious appetizer. There are over 350 different species of squid.

Trout and Salmon

Called *masu,* trout belongs to the same family as salmon. The salmon—*sake* in Japanese (not to be confused with rice wine)—and *masu* are very much alike and often difficult to distinguish. Generally, dog salmon is identified as *sake* and most of the smaller varieties (less than 25 inches in length) are considered to be *masu.* While *sake* is always an upstream fish, many varieties of *masu* are freshwater fish.

Both fish are highly esteemed in Japanese cuisine. Salmon caught in the sea is more popular than river salmon. Freshwater trout, on the other hand, is more appreciated than saltwater trout.

A 3½-ounce serving of rainbow trout contains about 195

Calories: 21.5 grams of protein, no carbohydrate, and 11.4 grams of fat.

Tuna

Tuna, a relative of the mackerel family, is called *maguro*, and is probably the most popular of all fish for *sushi* and *sashimi*. It has red flesh, *akami;* rich, pale pink flesh around the belly, *toro;* and pink meat between *toro* and *akami* called *chu-toro*. The flesh around the belly is called *toro* only when it contains a large amount of fat and the color is pale pink. All three cuts are greatly treasured in *sushi* and *sashimi*. A warning note to weight-conscious people: A *toro* cut has more than twice the caloric content of an *akami* cut. Here is the nutritional breakdown of a 3½-ounce serving of these two cuts: *Akami:* 133 Calories, 28.3 grams of protein, 1.4 grams of fat, and a trace of carbohydrate. *Toro:* 322 Calories, 21.4 grams of protein, 24.6 grams of fat, and a trace of carbohydrate.

The skipjack tuna family, *katsuo*, includes the ever-popular and important bonito. Bonito flakes are an essential ingredient in making *dashi*, the basic soup and cooking stock. *Katsuo* is best in the spring as a *sashimi* called *tataki*. *Maguro* is best in winter.

Yellowtail

Yellowtail, another fish that belongs to the same order as tuna but to a different family, is one of the most prized foods. The full-grown yellowtail, over 35 inches in length, is called *buri*. The smaller one, 30 to 35 inches long, is called *hamachi*. The full-grown fish are usually grilled. The best way to eat *hamachi* is raw in *sushi* and *sashimi*. The smaller yellowtails are called *warasa, inada,* and *wakashi*.

SHELLFISH—SEAFOOD NUMBER 2

Shellfish can be eaten raw or cooked, although certain kinds are usually precooked to a certain degree. Most shellfish help in a weight-control diet because they have a low caloric content and high-protein values. It all depends on the way each is served. Some shellfish, unfortunately, have a relatively high cholesterol content and must be consumed with care by those with cholesterol problems.

Clams

Each variety of clam has a different name and reputation. A typical raw cherrystone clam has the following nutritional breakdown. Four or five raw clams contain 56 Calories: 7.8 grams of protein, 4.1 grams of carbohydrate, and 0.6 gram of fat. Six clams, about 4½ ounces of seafood, contain 102 Calories: 14 grams of protein, 7.4 grams of carbohydrate, and 1.1 grams of fat. A 4-ounce serving of abalone contains 110 Calories: 20.9 grams of protein, 3.8 grams of carbohydrate, and no fat. Four ounces of scallops contain 91 Calories: 17.1 grams of protein, 3.7 grams of carbohydrate, and 0.2 gram of fat.

Here are the eight most popular types of Japanese clams:

- *Abalone: Awabi* is peachy to grayish in color. A favorite of West Coast residents, it is very chewy.
- *Ark shell:* Called *akagai,* this is the ark-shell clam or pepitona clam. Peachy to reddish in color, it is generally imported to the United States frozen.
- *Cockle: Torigai* is the cockle, black and white in color and very chewy.
- *Horseneck: Mirugai* is also called the horse-

neck clam, or geoduck. It is light peach in color. The long neck is usually eaten raw.
- *Pismo Beach: Hamaguri* is the Pismo Beach clam, another West Coast delight.
- *Red clam: Aoyagi* is actually orange in color, although it is called the "red" clam. It is usually parboiled before being served. It resembles the American quahog clam.
- *Scallop, large: Kaibashira* is also called *tairagai,* the large scallop.
- *Scallop, small: Kobashira* is light gold in color. This is the name for the succulent muscle that opens and closes the great clam.

Crab

Usually called *kani,* but also known as *gani,* the crab comes in eight hundred varieties. It is traditionally eaten cooked. It is also a popular seafood used in many types of salad. A 4-ounce serving of canned crab meat provides 113 Calories. Steamed, a 3½-ounce serving of crab meat contains about 92 Calories: 17 grams of protein, 0.5 gram of carbohydrate, and 1.9 grams of fat.

Oyster

Called *kaki,* the oyster is considered best eaten raw, although it can be served cooked. Six medium-sized oysters provide about 75 Calories. On the other hand, a cup of oyster stew, with milk, contains about 275 Calories. Three and a half ounces of raw oyster contain 67 Calories: 8.4 grams of protein, 3.5 grams of carbohydrate, and 2 grams of fat.

Shrimp

In Japanese, shrimp, jumbo shrimp, prawns, and sometimes lobster are usually lumped into the same category, *ebi*. The common Japanese shrimp and the red shrimp are usually eaten raw. But the flesh of shrimp can also be dried and pounded and served in many different ways.

Ama-ebi is shrimp, pink in color, eaten raw as a *sushi* delicacy. When the Japanese eat shrimp alive, it is called *odori;* which translates as "dance," meaning the shrimp is beheaded, shelled, and gutted so quickly that it is still moving when it is eaten.

Shrimp is the key seafood in cooking recipes, notably *tempura* (deep-fried shrimp), *teppan yaki* (grilled shrimp), and *teriyaki* (marinated shrimp). The Japanese believe, as does James Beard: "The unpardonable fault in preparing shrimp is overcooking."

Like other shellfish, shrimp is a low-Calorie food: when boiled, five large shrimp provide about 70 Calories. However, when fried, five large shrimp contain more than 300 Calories. The nutritional breakdown is as follows:

A 3½-ounce serving of ordinary boiled shrimp contains 107 Calories: 23 grams of protein and traces of carbohydrate and fat.

A 3½-ounce serving of fresh-fried shrimp contains 224 Calories: 20.3 grams of protein, 10 grams of carbohydrate, and 11 grams of fat.

That's quite a difference!

SEAWEED—SEAFOOD NUMBER 3

Seaweed is difficult to obtain in the United States as a foodstuff, although it can be purchased at certain health-food stores and in areas where the population eats Japanese-type food, as on the West Coast.

Seaweed is an especially important ingredient of *dashi*, the Japanese soup stock, as said before. But it can be served as a side dish too, or even in parts of a main course. It can also appear in various salad mixtures and other vegetable dishes.

Basically an algae, seaweed is a type of vegetation that can be divided into three main groups—green, red, and brown. Although there are many varieties of seaweed used in Japanese cooking, the most popular are four main types: *hijiki, kombu, nori,* and *wakame.*

Hijiki

Blackish and dried, this sea vegetation resembles licorice. It is usually cooked in *dashi* with other vegetables. Soaked in warm water before using, it takes getting used to.

Kombu

This is brown algae, usually dried cultivated kelp or sea tangle, primarily used as an active ingredient in the Japanese stock *dashi.* It can also serve as a vegetable dish, for *sushi* recipes, or for *sunomono* recipes. Shredded *kombu* can be used in soup and sautéed dishes. It can even be made into a tea-like beverage.

Nori

Even though *nori* is usually referred to as a red seaweed, it is technically laver, a kind of sea vegetation. It is usually marketed dried in a thin greenish-black sheet about 6 to 10 inches square. These sheets can be used as they are to wrap up *sushi. Nori* can also be crisped by being placed briefly over dry heat (electric stove or charcoal, but not gas, which produces a lot of moisture), and then crumbled over foods as a garnish for added flavor.

Wakame

This is dried sea vegetation, used mainly for salads and soups. It comes in long, curly strands. When soaked, the leaves open up. *Wakame*, like many other seaweeds, should always be soaked before using—at least for most dishes.

There are other types of seaweed, notably *mozuku* and *miru* (thick-haired codium), which hairlike seaweeds served mainly in *sunomono*, a type of Japanese salad. Generally speaking, of all foods seaweeds are the most free of Calories and the richest in minerals and vitamins.

Chapter 8

SUSHI AND *SASHIMI:*
EATING RAW

One of the most startling Japanese dishes—at least to most Americans—is fresh seafood, that is, fish and shellfish that are served *raw*. Although to the Western palate raw fish is not really an accepted delicacy, the practice of eating raw fish has spread around the world from Japan, and is now almost a familiar phenomenon in some American cities.

In the public mind, the word *sushi* has come to be associated with the consumption of raw fish, although there are really two words that should be associated with it—*sushi* and *sashimi*. Each describes the serving of fresh seafood in a different manner.

Sushi can be a full meal in itself; *sashimi* is usually served as a second or third course of a meal. To be a little more specific: Fresh seafood, sliced and decorated and placed on top of a rice patty as the main part of a meal, is called *sushi;* fresh seafood, served in a bowl or in a dish as part of a meal, is called *sashimi*.

Let's take *sashimi* first.

Sashimi

Sashimi is considered a Japanese delicacy rather than an hors d'oeuvre, which it might be considered by an American. It usually appears as sliced raw fish served with a little shredded seaweed, radish, or other vegetable.

The slices of flesh are arranged artistically against the shredded seaweed, lettuce, or radish to resemble a fish swimming through a deep, clear pool or creek. Part of the fun of eating *sashimi* is in seeing the arrangement first, then enjoying the flavor of the fresh fish and the vegetables that surround it.

Usually the diner dips the *sashimi* into a small saucer of *shoyu* mixed with *wasabi,* hot horseradish. To the surprise of most Westerners, *sashimi* does not smell like dead fish; that is only an ingrained prejudice that tends to put many people's backs up against eating *sashimi.*

Nor is the horseradish or mustard sauce served along with *sashimi* used to disguise the smell; rather, it is used to accentuate the flavor of the raw fish, which is very delicate and bland to the palate.

Sashimi is not confined to raw fish or shellfish. Although some of the best *sashimi* is composed of shrimp, prawns, and oysters, and sea bass, tuna, and swordfish, raw chicken meat can be served in the same manner.

The best time to eat *sashimi* with any meal is in the autumn or winter. Naturally, if you are thinking about serving it, be sure to purchase the best fresh fish you can, and serve it while it is still fresh!

Sushi

Although *sushi* can be properly thought of as part of a full meal, it is still considered by the Japanese as a type of snack food—not really an appetizer or hors d'oeuvre, but in essence something equivalent to a hamburger, a hot dog, or a pizza.

The key element in *sushi* is the vinegared rice. The garnishes (or ingredients) for *sushi* are not necessarily restricted to raw fish. They can be vegetables, eggs, cooked fish, or combinations of them. The garnishes can be mixed with rice, placed on top of rectangular rice patties or other shapes, rolled with rice, or even made into an envelope for stuffing with rice.

Three different types of *sushi* are the most common: *norimaki, chirashi,* and *nigiri.* What makes them differ is the form of preparation (rolled, simply mixed, or made into patties, etc.).

- *Norimaki-zushi:* The vinegared rice is spread on a sheet of edible seaweed called *nori,* then cooked ingredients, like sliced mushrooms, mashed fish, cooked eggs, and spinach, are placed at the center of the rice, and the entire sheet is rolled up.
- *Chirashi-zushi:* The vinegared rice is heaped in individual *donburi,* or bowls, then carefully and artistically dressed with bits of seasoned fried *tofu,* fish and shellfish, cooked egg, water chestnuts, and so on, and sliced ginger.
- *Nigiri-zushi:* This is composed of vinegared rice balls or ovals upon which the raw fish or shellfish is placed. *Wasabi* is placed between the rice and fish. This type of *sushi* is the most popular one in Tokyo today.

Japanese use the term "rice sandwiches" to describe *nigiri-zushi* to Americans. The rice serves as the bread and the raw seafood as the sandwich ingredient, as explained above.

In Tokyo there are literally hundreds of *sushi* restaurants or shops—called *sushi* bars—located all over town. In fact, the reason the *sushi* shop is called a bar is that it resembles the old frontier bars popular in Western fiction (and reality).

The long, narrow shop is divided in the middle by a counter of cypress wood—just like a bar—behind which the *sushi* chef works. In front of the counter sits the customer. Half the fun in a *sushi* bar is watching the chef perform after the customer has indicated his choice of fish.

At the chef's elbow stands a wooden tub filled with vinegared rice prepared beforehand. On the top of the counter sit bottles of *shoyu* and bowls of sliced ginger. After the order is given, the chef scoops up a handful of rice, shapes it deftly into a smooth ball or oval, selects a razor-sharp knife, and cuts the fish chosen, placing it on top of the rice patty.

He then puts the *sushi* on a lacquer tray with an arrangement of palm or green leaves, or some such imaginative display. Along with the *sushi* comes a cup of hot tea served in a large cup. The customer may opt to drink a glass of cold beer in the Western fashion.

To eat *sushi* the diner lifts the "sandwich" in the fingers, dips it in a bowl of *shoyu* nearby, and eats it—probably in one bite. What the amateur *sushi* eater must avoid is dipping the rice part of the sandwich into the sauce; it is the fish part only that should be dunked. Otherwise, the fish will slip off the rice patty.

In addition to having a cypress counter, most *sushi* bars are designed to resemble an old-style Japanese country cottage. Most have small tables near the bar along with the stools that serve customers who prefer to sit at the counter.

Old *sushi* hands like to sit at the bar and order individual pieces of fish as their fancy dictates. These are displayed in a glass-topped case—live prawns, squid, octopus, tuna, and white-fleshed fish like flounder, sea bass, sea bream, clams, abalone, and scallops.

SUSHI AS A MAIN COURSE

The frequenter of the *sushi* bar eats *sushi* more or less as a snack. However, *sushi* can be eaten as the main course of a dinner. In that case, it may be served with a first course—something cooked, steamed, or grilled. Then a type of salad—spinach with sesame sauce, for example—can be added to the dinner, to be topped off with a delicate clear soup.

Nigiri-zushi, today the most popular type of *sushi,* was developed in Tokyo in the early nineteenth century. It was invented as a very early form of fast-food service—to accommodate theatergoers watching Kabuki shows. The idea was for the patrons of the Kabuki to sneak out just before the third act to grab a snack before going back to see the end of the play. In that early version of *sushi,* there was no elaboration of service—only quick forming of the rice balls, quick slicing of the fish, and quick service.

The word *sushi* comes from *su,* which at present means "vinegar," and *shi,* which means to "control" or to "arrange." Actually, vinegar is a very modern reading of the Japanese character for *su. Su* comes from the Chinese *ju,* which originally meant "long life," or something to that effect.

VARIATIONS ON THE *SUSHI* THEME

There are special variations of *sushi* that give it versatility and long life. In one variant, the chef cuts a square of seaweed, coats it quickly with rice, then places seafood or some other item in the middle of the rice. He then coats the whole with *wasabi,* and the seaweed is rolled into a cylinder that can be cut into pieces or eaten as is.

Whatever foodstuff is inside the cylinder gives the name to the type of *sushi.* If it is an omelet of fish and egg, the *sushi* is called *date maki.* If fresh tuna is placed inside, it is called *tekka maki.* If the inner food is cooked dried gourd, it is called *nori maki*. If it is cucumber, it is called *kappa maki*. (*Maki* means "a roll.")

Using the same base, the chef can roll it up on the bias to form a shape exactly like an American ice-cream cone. The shaped *sushi* is called *temaki-zushi*.

Another variant is vinegared rice in a bag made of fried *tofu*, called *inari-zushi*. Still another is vinegared rice wrapped in bamboo leaves, called *sasa maki zushi*. If seafood is scattered over a bowl of vinegared rice, the dish becomes *chirashi-zushi*.

THE MOST POPULAR TYPES OF RAW SEAFOOD FOR *SUSHI*

A number of the best-known and loved *nigiri-zushi* dishes in Japan are the following (these names refer to the raw seafood that makes up the *sushi*):

- *Akagai:* ark-shell *sushi*
- *Anago:* grilled conger-eel *sushi*
- *Awabi:* abalone *sushi*
- *Buri:* yellowtail *sushi*
- *Chu-toro:* *sushi* made from the side section of the tuna
- *Ebi:* *sushi* made from boiled or live shrimp
- *Hamachi:* *sushi* made from the very young yellowtail
- *Ika:* squid *sushi*
- *Ikura:* salmon-roe *sushi*
- *Maguro:* tuna *sushi*
- *Tai:* sea-bream *sushi*
- *Tako:* octopus *sushi*
- *Toro:* *sushi* made from the underside of the tuna
- *Uni:* sea-urchin *sushi*

You can even put thick, sweet omelet on rice to produce a very special *sushi—tamago yaki!*

SUSHI IN A WEIGHT-CONSCIOUS DIET

A glance at the caloric and protein values in the section on seafood will give you the primary reason for opting for *sushi* over other fast-food delicacies like hamburgers, pizzas, and fried chicken in a basket.

Most fresh fish have a very low caloric content per ounce of serving; the combination of low Calories and high protein makes fish and seafood the most valuable source of nutrients for the healthy person. Because rice, the major constituent of *sushi*, is a bulky food that gives a sensation of fullness or satisfaction, the combination of rice and raw fish is conducive to excellent weight control.

The only thing to watch out for is the use of too much *shoyu*, or soy sauce. Soy sauce, as has been mentioned, has a very high sodium content. However, only a drop of soy sauce is enough to enjoy *sushi*. You just have to practice eating it so that your pieces do not soak up too much soy sauce.

PART THREE:

Sayonara to Fat!

Chapter 9

COOKING THAT LIMITS WEIGHT

Unlike Americans, the Japanese basically plan their menus according to the natural seasons of the year. The themes of the various seasons are accentuated not only by the selection of food and type of cooking, but also by the decorative arrangements of the vegetables, meat, and seafood.

There are a number of fundamental concepts in Japanese meal planning. Once you understand them, you will find that there are infinite variations possible for the imaginative cook.

Here are a dozen of the most important ideas in Japanese menu organization:

Rice

Rice is served at every Japanese meal except when noodles or another rice dish becomes the main course. The rice is practically always served hot and plain. It is also always cooked in the traditional manner, with almost no variation.

Soup

Soup is served at almost every Japanese meal. There are basically only two kinds: *misoshiru* and *sumashi jiru*. The ingredients are of course limitless. Generally, soup is not served first, but it may come either before the main course or after it.

Pickles

Pickles—called *tsukemono*—are served at almost every meal, usually with a bowl of hot rice. Japanese pickles are unlike Western pickles. (See discussion later in this chapter.)

Dishes

As mentioned above, the Japanese pay particular attention to the seasons in planning menus. Most vegetables and seafood are served in season when they are most plentiful and fresh. The selection of vegetables and seafoods depends on what is available in quantity and quality. The type of preparation also varies with the season.

Winter dishes: During the winter, most meals are built around hot dishes. These include meals cooked in one pot, with the guests dipping in and eating food hot from the source. This type of cuisine is called *nabemono* cooking. (See discussion below.)

Summer dishes: During the summer, most meals are built around cold or room-temperature dishes. These include meals of cold noodles, *sushi, sashimi,* chilled *sunomono* (vinegared salad), and pickles.

Another important point in the selection of dishes is that most Japanese cooks plan to have only one so-called main dish. When serving *sukiyaki* or *tempura,* for example, they prepare side dishes ahead of time to be served at room temperature. Then during the meal, they can concentrate on cooking the main dish.

Sauces

The Japanese cook usually tries to vary the monotony of the sauces and marinades used in a meal. If the main dish is flavored with soy sauce, side dishes might be flavored with *miso* dressing or a *dashi* broth.

Foodstuffs

Not only should sauces and marinades be varied from dish to dish, but the foodstuffs should also be varied. If fish is the main dish, chicken or shrimp might be served as the appetizer.

Cooking Methods

In turn, the Japanese cook plans to use different kinds of cooking methods in preparing the various dishes. There are many different ways to prepare foods in Japanese cuisine. A full discussion follows later in this chapter.

Service

In serving food, the Japanese cook usually tries to keep each dish separate, believing that individual flavorings and characteristics should be maintained.

Beverages

Most Japanese meals end with a beverage of some kind— usually green tea. However, *sake* or white wine can be served with any meal. Tea, called *cha* in Japanese, is usually drunk last, after the remaining bits of rice are finished off, but sometimes can be served during the meal, as at a *sushi* bar.

THIRTEEN VARIATIONS ON BASIC COOKING METHODS

The Japanese have special words to classify the type of dish based on the method used to cook or prepare it. Most of these methods are familiar to the average American. As mentioned earlier, there are two especially important types of cooking missing from the typical Japanese cuisine: baking and roasting.

The reason has to do with Japanese cooking methods and utensils. Usually, a closed oven is not used, but the food is cooked in pots over a direct flame or on a skewer over a direct flame or heat. Thus, baking and roasting, which require a closed heating element, are usually excluded.

In present-day Japan, of course, many Tokyo citizens do have ovens much like those Americans have. However, most traditional Japanese dishes do not include baking or roasting. Actually, even a broiled dish is usually grilled in typical Japanese cuisine.

Here are thirteen different categories of dishes, based on the types of preparation and the Japanese names for each. A brief explanation of Japanese beverages is also given.

Aemono

An *aemono* dish is composed of a mixture of raw or cooked vegetables, fish, or cooked meats, or combinations of these with a sauce of some kind. The sauce is usually rather thick, and sometimes it is poured over the other ingredients.

SAYONARA TO FAT!

Agemono

An *agemono* dish is a preparation of vegetables and/or meats fried in vegetable oil. There are two main frying methods: *tempura* and *kara-age*.

- *Tempura:* The *tempura* method of frying is used with seafood and vegetables that first have been dipped in batter and then are immersed in deep oil and fried. Unlike in Western-style deep frying, the vegetables and seafood are not left long in the oil so that very little oil is absorbed by them.
- *Kara-age:* The *kara-age* method of frying is used with seafood, meat, or vegetables that first are lightly dusted with cornstarch and then are fried in deep, hot vegetable oil. Again, the foods are not left in the frying pan as long as Western fried foods are, and the amount of fat used is much less than that used in Western cooking.

Gohanmono

A *gohanmono*, or *meshimono*, dish is one whose base is rice. This includes seasoned rice, *donburimono*, and even many types of *sushi*, although *sushi* is often treated separately. The simplest form of *gohanmono* is the plain white rice served with practically every Japanese meal.

Menrui

A *menrui* dish is a serving of noodles. It can be in a separate dish, or it can be combined with sauce or other condiments. *Menrui* is a typical lunch dish in Tokyo.

Mushimono

A *mushimono* dish is food steamed in a container placed over another (and covered) pot, or in a pan holding steaming water. The food to be steamed is usually a combination of vegetables, a piece of meat, an egg, fish, or shellfish. A favorite *mushimono* dish is *chawanmushi,* an egg dish of custardlike consistency, containing some vegetables and seafood.

Nabemono

A *nabemono* dish is a very important type of cooking in Japan. It is prepared in one pot or saucepan for an entire assembly of guests. *Nabemono,* in fact, usually refers to saucepan cooking or stir-fry cooking at the table. One typical *nabemono* dish is *sukiyaki,* composed of mixed vegetables plus beef or poultry. *Sukiyaki* is the most popular of all *nabemono* dishes, and is quite well known in America. There are others:

- *Mizutaki,* boiled chicken, is also a familiar *nabemono* dish. Chicken and vegetables are boiled in a pot in front of the guests, who take out portions as they become ready and dip them in a *ponzu* sauce, a mixture of soy sauce and the juice of a type of citrus fruit.
- *Shabu-shabu* is a variety of *mizutaki.* Paper-thin slices of meat are dipped in a boiling broth with a pair of chopsticks and stirred to cook very quickly—in several seconds—and then eaten with a sauce the way *mizutaki* is eaten. *"Shabu-shabu"* represents the sound made by stirring the broth with a piece of meat. There is a variety of sauces—every family or restaurant has its own special recipe for *shabu-shabu* sauce. Invent your own!

Vegetables are also included in this dish, just like *mizutaki.*

- *Yosenabe* is another dish in which the ingredients are cooked in a broth. The broth is usually slightly seasoned with soy sauce and *sake.* This dish features an assortment *(yose)* of seafood—usually white-meat fish and types of clams, shrimp, and crabs—cooked together with vegetables such as *tofu,* bamboo shoots, *shiitake,* and crown daisy.

In *nabemono* dining the guests sit around the saucepan watching its contents simmer in the middle of the table. An electric saucepan is a very handy appliance for preparing a *nabemono* dinner. (See fuller discussion later in the chapter.)

Nimono

A *nimono* dish is a food or group of foods cooked in a seasoned liquid. This dish vaguely resembles a kind of Western stew. *Nimono* is different because of the nature of the seasoned liquid used to flavor it, and it is usually served with a small amount of cooking liquid. The Japanese use *dashi,* to which have been added *shoyu, mirin,* or *miso.* A *nimono* dish can include vegetables, seafood, or meat. The seasoning can also be accentuated by adding vegetable oil or a bit of ginger, Japanese pepper, or red pepper. In a variation of *nimono,* the food is first lightly fried, then boiled for a short time, then sprinkled with a few drops of seasoning oil such as sesame oil.

Sashimi

A *sashimi* dish is always composed of raw fish, sliced, and served as is, as described in Chapter 8.

NOTE: *This* is the type of dish Americans think of as *sushi*.

Shirumono

A *shirumono* dish is a soup—all soups fall in this category. Soup is served at almost every Japanese meal. Two of the most important types are *miso* soup and *sumashi* soup. *Miso* soup is basically a bouillon seasoned with *miso*. It contains some vegetables and perhaps meat or seafood. *Sumashi* soup, clear soup, is a bouillon seasoned mainly with salt and soy sauce. It too contains some seafood, meat, or egg together with vegetables.

Sunomono

A *sunomono* dish is a kind of mixed salad seasoned with a rice-vinegar dressing. The ingredients of a typical *sunomono* can be predominantly vegetables, usually mixed, and/or seafood of various kinds, or even fruits.

Sushi

A *sushi* dish is a combination of a food of some kind and rice flavored with vinegar.

NOTE: Many *sushi* dishes involve rice mixed with uncooked fish. The popular American concept of *sushi* is that it is generally a raw-fish dish. The real meaning of the word is something else, and it usually indicates the use of a rice patty on which the raw fish is placed. (Chapter 8 covers the story of *sushi* and *sashimi*.)

Tsukemono

The word *tsukemono* is a general term for pickled food. Japanese pickles are quite different from American pickles, and in a sense they are an important foodstuff, appearing at almost every meal. There are six basic types of pickled vegetables, differentiated according to the pickling agent used: salt, *miso*, *nuka*, *sake* lees, *koji*, and vinegar.

Salt: When salt is used, the pickling is accomplished by pressure and fermentation, giving the vegetable its special crispy texture and tart taste.

Miso: When *miso*, fermented soybean paste, is used, the process is known as *misozuke*. This type of pickling takes place in a bed of *miso*.

Nuka: *Nuka* is rice bran, the fine skin removed from brown rice during the polishing process. Pickling by *nuka* is called *nukamiso-zuke*, and is the method favored all over Japan for home pickling. In the process, *nuka* is mixed with water and salt and then allowed to ferment. To this base other condiments or spices such as red-hot pepper, mustard, ginger, and so on, are added to give the pickle its distinctive flavor. When the *nuka* fermentation bed is ready, the vegetables are put in it to pickle anywhere from overnight to several weeks.

Sake lees: The mash left over after *sake* has been manufactured is composed of *sakekasu*, or *sake* lees. A bed of this mixture is used to pickle vegetables in a process called *kasuzuke*.

Koji: *Koji* is a mixture of steamed rice, barley, or soybeans that has been combined with a type of mold. In pickling, *koji* is made into a pickling bed, and vegetables are incubated in it. The process is called *kojizuke*.

Vinegar: The pickling vinegar in Japan is white vinegar made from rice. Vinegar pickles are usually of two different kinds: *gari*, or pickled ginger, and *rakkyo*. *Gari* is commonly served with *sushi*. *Rakkyo* is a kind of scallionlike bulb (shallot).

Yakimono

A *yakimono* dish involves grilled foods, like seafood or meat. However, the dish can easily include vegetables—even fruit—along with chicken and small birds. The grilling is usually done directly over a charcoal fire, with the foods spitted on a skewer. The Japanese *konro*—similar to a Western barbecue grill—is generally used for *yakimono*.

There are three different types of grilling:

- *Shioyaki:* This type of grilling means that salt is used as one of the chief ingredients in preparing the food for grilling.
- *Flavor grilling:* This type of grilling involves brushing the food with a mixture of *shoyu*, *mirin*, or *dashi* to marinate it as it is being grilled. Two favorite flavor-grilled Japanese dishes are *yakitori* (broiled chicken) and *teriyaki* (fish marinated in a sauce containing *shoyu*).
- *Miso grilling:* This type of grilling is used to prepare vegetables like eggplant and some seafood and meat dishes as well.

Beverages

The main Japanese alcoholic beverage is *sake* (also called *nihon shu*). It is served with the meal, or, what is more likely, rice and pickles are served at the end, and the dishes that go well with *sake* come first. In Japan today, white wine and beer quite often accompany the meal.

The main Japanese nonalcoholic beverage is, of course, tea. Practically all Japanese meals end with tea. The following are some of the important varieties used:

- *Bancha:* green tea for everyday use
- *Genmaicha:* tea flavored with roasted rice grains
- *Gyokuro:* very high-quality green tea
- *Hojicha:* roasted tea
- *Matcha:* powdered green tea. This is the tea used for the Japanese tea ceremony
- *Sencha:* high-quality green tea

NOTE: Remember one important thing about drinking tea the Japanese way:

Do not use sugar!

FACTS ABOUT THE PREPARATION OF JAPANESE FOOD

One important point about Japanese cooking—no matter what kind—is that a dish usually requires a maximum of time for preparation, serving, and eating . . . and a *minimum* of time for actual cooking.

This not only cuts down on the amount of valuable energy spent in preparing the food, but it also helps preserve natural flavors and nutrients.

The Japanese also spend a great deal more time than Americans do in washing and cutting up ingredients before they are put in a pot or pan for cooking. There are several good reasons for such careful cleaning. Since much of the food being prepared is almost ready for eating, it must be clean to the point where it can be eaten immediately. Cooking is not expected to boil away impurities or kill germs in the food. There is another important purpose in washing foodstuffs, particularly green vegetables with harsh tastes. By washing just-cooked green vegetables, the cook can eliminate harsh tastes and preserve their green—and fresh—appearance, enhancing their appeal. Since Japanese cuisine involves a minimum of cooking, the food, without embellishment, can look bright and immaculate and appetizing.

Because the Japanese eat their food with chopsticks, not forks, spoons, or knives, the chef usually cuts everything into bite-size portions before cooking or serving so it can be handled easily with chopsticks. This is true of vegetables served raw or uncooked, like spinach or cabbage. Meat and fish also must be cut into pieces that are easily managed with chopsticks.

Look what happens: By cutting fish and meat into small chunks before cooking, the amount of cooking time required is minimized.

FACTS ABOUT THE SERVING OF JAPANESE FOOD

Food is rarely served piping hot in Japan—as is the habit in the West—but at room temperature. This means that in hot weather, food can be prepared with a minimum of heat in the kitchen. It also means that the host or hostess does not have to hustle back and forth carrying in hot plates. The entire serving atmosphere is a more tranquil one, with both host(ess) and guests in a relaxed and calm frame of mind.

This in turn helps establish a genuine feeling of fellowship and conviviality, which, as every physician and nutritionist knows, puts the diner into the optimum condition for good tasting, good eating, and good digestion. A relaxed attitude at the table and a comfortable, unhectic pace of eating are conducive to a better-adjusted metabolism. This gives the diner psychological control over the amount of food he or she eats.

Serving food is as important as preparing it, according to Japanese custom. For example, the way in which each separate item is placed on the plate or plates creates an atmosphere of calm and artistic beauty that is beneficial in itself. The cook, having taken great care in cutting, washing, and cooking the food, now has the final pleasure of placing the food in front of the guest in its most appealing shape and form.

Psychologically the fulfillment of putting together a great meal can be attained only by the final display of the food before the guest. By now, the expertise and artistry of the cook has come to full flower. The placement of the food, the shapes and designs of the individual foodstuffs, the color and texture of the specific items—all contribute to the over-all image of the perfect meal.

Now the cook can realize the joy of success.

FACTS ABOUT THE EATING OF JAPANESE FOOD

At serving time the diner is in the position of maximum receptivity. Not only has the smell of cooking food whetted the appetite, but the careful and picturesque placement of the food items on the plates has maximized expectation to the utmost. Now the point of all this painstaking food preparation becomes evident. The diner knows that great care has been taken in the cooking and determines in turn that great care will also be taken in its eating.

It is a fact that a person who eats too rapidly will probably overeat. The digestion and absorption of food start soon after the first mouthful is taken. When a certain amount of nutrients have been absorbed in the system, a signal is sent to the brain that bodily needs have been fulfilled. Satisfaction thus is registered inside the body. And the meal ends.

If for any reason the diner eats too swiftly, more than enough food will be taken in before the signal of fulfillment can reach the brain to stop eating. Obviously a person who eats too rapidly will eat too much. Also, if someone eats fast foods all the time, the habit of overeating will persist, causing additional weight problems.

For psychologically perfect dining, the diner must be in a relaxed and calm mood. Certainly it does not hurt to see in front of you a nicely designed, artistic dish, placed on colorful or intricately designed plates and ready for contemplative eating.

FACTS ABOUT THE ENJOYMENT OF JAPANESE FOOD

There is a series of definite positive results from experiencing such a mood of contentment:

- The diner handles the food as carefully and as delicately as the cook did when preparing it.
- The diner puts small pieces of food into the mouth for easier digestion.
- With a leisurely pace established at the outset, the diner uses eating utensils carefully from beginning to end and does not use fingers to bolt down food à la Henry VIII.
- For the best possible gratification of the taste buds, the diner eats only one kind of food at a time. Mixing items that have been carefully prepared separately destroys the flavor of each.
- The diner savors the taste of each food in the mouth and chews it carefully, allowing its taste to penetrate the palate.
- As the taste stimulates the palate, the diner experiences all the joys of gourmet eating, and is most receptive to its gastronomic pleasures.

- Naturally the more slowly a diner chews food, the more easily and completely it will be digested, easing the physiological processes of the body and cutting down on gastric upsets and overindulgence.
- A slow eater generally does not eat as much as a fast eater. With the proper atmosphere set by the host or hostess, the diner enjoys the food much more.
- It is the slow eater who experiences a gourmet's pleasure. No one who considers himself or herself a gourmet will ruin the joy of eating by ingesting food too rapidly.

THE JAPANESE ORDER OF DINNER DISHES

Roughly speaking, there are two formal ways of serving food in Japan:

- One way is called *kuikiri*, which closely resembles Western custom. The first course is brought to the table. When finished, the empty dish is then removed and the second course brought in, and so on.
- The other way is to serve several courses at once on a small individual table in front of each diner. When the diner finishes eating what is on the table, it is removed and a second table with more dishes is substituted. At a very elaborate dinner, three or even four tables are used.

In any case, these two serving methods are used in restaurants or at very formal meals; the average Japanese family does not eat or serve dinner every day in the home this way.

At a family-type meal, practically everything is laid out on the table. Rice, soup, *sashimi*, broiled dish, and steamed dishes are usually presented individually. Pickles and other condiments are often placed in a big bowl or plate to be selected by each diner according to preference. *Sunomono, aemono,* and *nimono* can be served either individually or in a big bowl for everyone.

When guests are invited to a Japanese home, the way food is served will be a compromise between restaurant style and casual style, depending on the intimacy, relationship, occasion, personality of the host or hostess and guests, facility, type of food to be served, and so on.

When several dishes are served at once, the Japanese usually eat the hot foods first. The rice is continually nibbled, especially at a dinner where no *sake* is served. It is also always the very last thing to be finished before tea.

The main course is eaten somewhere in the middle of the meal, although it may be placed anywhere and in any order. Vegetables, either in the form of cooked dishes or fresh salads, are usually included and placed around the main dish. In some cases, both salads and cooked vegetables surround the main course.

With tea, the dessert is usually served. It can consist of fresh fruit slices, or even sweetened cakes and small confections made from red beans, rice, and agar-agar (a gelatin derived from seaweed), millet jelly (a cereal grain like barley, ground into gruel), eggs, and sugar, enhanced with aromatic flavoring and attractive colorings.

ENDLESS VARIATIONS ON THE MAIN THEME

As for the main course in the Japanese dinner, the varieties are as endless as the main course of a Western meal can be. For example, you can serve beef and poultry, although the Japanese do not eat as much of these meats as Westerners do. Or you can serve fish or shellfish, always popular in Tokyo.

In addition to the various types of foodstuffs served, they can be prepared in different ways, as we have seen already: boiling, broiling, frying, deep frying, stir-frying, steaming, grilling, in almost every way except roasting and baking.

EATING OUT OF THE SAUCEPAN

A word about *nabemono:* The word usually refers to stir-fried or "saucepan" foods that are prepared in front of the diners so that each can lift food right out of the saucepan and onto the plate immediately without time wasted in serving.

In *nabemono* the food is always cut ahead of time into bite-size pieces and cooked in a broth that bubbles in a pot on a brazier or hot plate. Today, many *nabemono* meals are cooked in an electric saucepan in the middle of the table.

Because of the intimate atmosphere created by *nabemono* cooking, a Japanese host or hostess often serves this type of dish for close friends or for rather casual dinner parties. Since most of the *nabemono* menu includes some animal protein like poultry, meat, and fish as well as a variety of vegetables, and is often cooked in broth, one *nabemono* dish will replace soup, main dish, and vegetable dish. Besides, it is always cooked at the table, and the host or hostess does not have to run back and forth between the dining room and the kitchen.

A typical *nabemono* dinner should include an hors d'oeuvre, a *nabemono*, rice, a pickled vegetable, and a light dessert.

Chapter 10

KEEP-THE-POUNDS-DOWN RECIPES

The following selection of recipes comprises all dishes marked with an * in the seven menus in Chapter 3 and in the fifteen-day menus in Chapter 12. It also encompasses many Japanese dishes that are traditional and that are guaranteed to be good combinations to help keep weight down. Some dishes also are not typically Japanese.

In the selection of the recipes, particular attention has been paid to the availability of certain items, and possible substitutions have been included if a Japanese item is hard to find. Also, special sauces, dips, and garnishes are made a part of the recipe for which they have been created. Many popular Japanese dishes may be missing from the selection, but this book is not intended to be a cookbook.

This chapter is divided into the following sections:

- Basic stocks: These are various soup stocks normally used.
- Soups: These are both clear and thick soups, plus variations.
- Salads: These recipes feature some of the more popular Japanese vegetable items.

- Vegetables: These include recipes for sauces as well as vegetable combinations.
- *Sushi* and *sashimi* dishes
- *Tofu* dishes
- Fruit dishes
- Main dishes: These include several dishes arranged according to the featured ingredient: beef, seafood, fish, chicken, and egg.

Basic Stocks

Dashi 1 (Ichiban dashi)

NOTE: The two most widely used kinds of *dashi*, the basic stock in Japanese cooking, serve as a soup base and as a liquid ingredient in many dishes. If it is impossible to procure any of the recipe items listed, you can always substitute chicken stock or vegetable stock.

	4- to 5-inch-square *kombu* (sea vegetation)
5	cups water
½	scant cup flaked *katsuobushi* (dried bonito flakes)

Wash *kombu* thoroughly and place in a saucepan together with water. Bring water to boil and remove *kombu*. Add *katsuobushi* to broth, remove from burner immediately, and let steep a minute or two. Strain the liquid through clean cheesecloth or a fine strainer. Save *katsuobushi* and *kombu* for preparing *dashi 2*.

Dashi 2 (Niban dashi)

katsuobushi saved from *dashi 1*
kombu saved from *dashi 1*

3 cups water
(⅓ cup flaked *katsuobushi*, optional)

Put *katsuobushi* and *kombu* in a saucepan together with water. Bring to a boil, let simmer for several minutes, and remove from burner. Strain the liquid through cheesecloth. Discard *katsuobushi* and *kombu*.

NOTE: When a strong stock is desired, add extra *katsuobushi*.

Chicken stock

2 to 3 pounds chicken bones (necks, legs, backs, wings)
12 to 15 cups water

Make some cracks on the long bones with the back of a chef's knife. Combine bones and water in a large kettle and bring to boil. Skim off the impurity when broth starts to boil. Let simmer uncovered about 3 hours. Strain through cheesecloth. Discard bones. Skim off all fat. The yield will be about 5 to 6 cups clear chicken stock.

Vegetable stock

Place leftover vegetables, vegetable parings, and some cut-up fresh vegetables in a pot with ample water. Simmer uncovered about 3 hours. Strain. Discard vegetables.

Soups

Miso soup
Serves 4

½   to 1 cup of solid ingredients of
your choice, such as potatoes,
zucchini, carrots, turnips, scallions,
etc., cut into small pieces

3⅓   cups *dashi 1* or *2* or vegetable
stock*

4   tablespoons medium-salty *miso*

OR

3   tablespoons dark, strong salty *miso*

Cook solid ingredients in the *dashi* until tender. Place small
quantity of *dashi* in a bowl and dissolve *miso* in it. Then pour
dissolved *miso* into the simmering *dashi* with solids. Bring to
a simmer again, but do not allow to boil. Ladle into individual soup bowls.

Clear soup
Serves 4

3¾   cups *dashi 1* or vegetable stock*

½   teaspoon salt

1½   teaspoons soy sauce

2   teaspoons *sake* or dry sherry
(optional)

     Solid ingredients of your choice
(parboiled spinach, sliced
mushrooms, or hard-boiled eggs
cut in half, etc.)

111

Combine *dashi*, salt, and soy sauce in a saucepan, and bring to boil. Add *sake* if desired. Remove from heat. In each soup bowl place small quantities of the solid ingredients of your choice, ready for consumption, such as parboiled spinach, sliced mushrooms, or hard-boiled eggs cut in half. Ladle the clear soup into the bowls, garnish with sprigs of parsley, diced scallions, or lemon-peel curls, and serve hot. Again, let your imagination be your guide as to garnishes.

Clear soup with chicken
Serves 4

½   chicken breast, cut into 8 bite-size pieces
¼   cup soy sauce
4   cups *dashi* or vegetable stock*
     salt
     sprigs of parsley

Boil chicken pieces in soy sauce until just tender. Put 2 pieces of chicken in each soup bowl. Bring vegetable stock or *dashi* to boil and adjust seasoning with salt and soy sauce in which chicken was cooked. Pour piping-hot vegetable stock or *dashi* over the chicken pieces and garnish each bowl with a sprig of parsley.

Japanese noodle *(soba)* soup
Serves 4

8   ounces *soba* (dry) buckwheat noodles
     about 2 quarts boiling water
2   pints *dashi 1* or chicken stock (well skimmed)

⅓   cup soy sauce
⅓   cup *mirin* (sweet white wine),
     white port, or cream sherry
¼   teaspoon salt
½   pound boneless chicken breast
     (skin removed), cut into bite-size
     pieces
3   scallion stalks, cut into 1-inch
     lengths

CONDIMENTS:

shredded *nori* (dry laver)
ground coriander seeds
shichimi-togarashi (seven-flavored
Japanese spice)

Cook *soba* in 2 quarts boiling water the same way you cook spaghetti (7 to 10 minutes). Drain *soba* well and cool under running water. Season stock or *dashi* with mixture of soy sauce, *mirin,* and salt, and bring to boil. Add chicken pieces when stock is boiling. Add scallions when chicken pieces are cooked. Add *soba* to boiling soup before serving to heat up the *soba.* Serve *soba* in *donburi* bowls and pour soup over them together with chicken and scallion pieces. Serve condiments separately.

Prawn and cucumber soup
Serves 6

½   pound prawns
1   cucumber
5   cups *dashi 1* or vegetable stock
6   sliced fresh mushrooms
1   tablespoon *sake,* dry white wine, or
     dry sherry

2   tablespoons soy sauce
¼   to ½ teaspoon salt
2   ounces turnip greens
½   teaspoon grated lemon peel

Shell and devein raw prawns and cut into thirds. Peel and quarter cucumber lengthwise. Remove seeds and cut into ½-inch lengths. Cut the turnip greens in ½-inch lengths. Bring *dashi* or stock to boil and add prawns, cucumber, and mushrooms. When prawns are cooked, add *sake*, soy sauce, salt, and turnip greens. Cook for another 1 to 2 minutes. Garnish with lemon peel and serve.

Egg drop soup
Serves 4

3½   cups *dashi 1* or chicken stock
½   teaspoon salt
2   teaspoons cornstarch
¼   cup cold water
2   eggs
      gingerroot

In a small bowl, dissolve cornstarch in cold water. Beat eggs in another bowl. In a saucepan, bring *dashi* or stock to boil, season with salt, and stir in cornstarch mixture until smooth. Bring to boil again. Slowly pour beaten eggs into stock in a thin stream and with a circular motion. The soup will be done when the egg floats to the top in threads. Pour into individual bowls. Add a dash of grated gingerroot to each bowl.

Salads

NOTE: Japanese salads are a combination of carefully selected ingredients, tossed with a sauce of white vinegar and soy sauce or salt, or a slightly thickened dressing flavored with *mirin,* soy sauce, lemon juice, sesame seeds, or *wasabi.*

Carrot *namasu*
Serves 6

½ pound *daikon,* white radishes, or turnips, cut into julienne strips
1 carrot, scraped and cut into julienne strips
1 teaspoon salt
1 teaspoon sugar
1 tablespoon white vinegar

Mix *daikon,* carrot, and salt in a large mixing bowl and let stand 30 minutes. Lightly wash and drain vegetables to eliminate excess salt, squeeze dry, and put into a clean bowl. Combine sugar and white vinegar, add to vegetables, and mix well. Serve at room temperature in small individual dishes as a salad course or as a condiment.

Cucumber and sesame seed salad
Serves 6

2 small cucumbers
salt
¼ cup lemon juice
½ teaspoon soy sauce
2 tablespoons toasted sesame seeds
1 cup flaked crab meat

Score cucumbers with fork to leave some dark green skin for color. Cut cucumbers in half and remove seeds. Slice each

115

cucumber half into thin diagonal slices. Place them in a mixing bowl and sprinkle with salt. Let stand about 30 minutes. Rinse slices in ice-cold water and squeeze out excess liquid. Place cucumber slices in bowl. Add remaining 4 ingredients and toss.

Daikon salad with shrimp
Serves 6

1	*daikon* (about the size of a medium cucumber)
½	tablespoon sugar
¼	cup mild vinegar
	pinch of salt
½	small cucumber, cubed
6	large cooked shrimp, diced
1	teaspoon freshly grated horseradish (not necessary if *daikon* is pungent)
1	teaspoon freshly grated gingerroot

Wash *daikon;* peel and grate fine. Lightly squeeze out excess liquid. In small bowl, combine sugar, vinegar, and salt, and mix well. Add to grated *daikon.* Mix dressed *daikon* with cubed cucumber, diced shrimp, horseradish, and gingerroot. Shape in mounds and serve on shredded lettuce or other salad greens.

NOTE: A fresh, ripe persimmon, diced slightly larger than the cucumber cubes, may be substituted for the cooked shrimp and sugar in this recipe. This combination is a great favorite in Japan during the fall, when fresh persimmons are available.

Spinach *sunomono*
Serves 4

½   pound spinach, washed

DRESSING:

½   teaspoon sugar
2   teaspoons rice vinegar (white vinegar)
2   teaspoons *sake* (optional)
1   teaspoon soy sauce

Parboil spinach in water until just barely tender. Cooking time should be very short. Rinse spinach in cold water, squeeze dry. Cut leaves and stems into 1-inch lengths.

DRESSING: In bowl, mix sugar, vinegar, *sake,* and soy sauce. Add spinach and toss to coat with dressing. Serve in small individual dishes.

Chinese cabbage in vinegar
Serves 4

3   Chinese cabbage leaves
3   cups water
2   tablespoons white vinegar
¼   teaspoon soy sauce
½   teaspoon sugar
    dried red-pepper flakes

Cabbage leaves should measure about 6 x 10 inches. If smaller, use additional leaves. Trim ragged edges and cut each leaf in half. Bring water to boil in a saucepan. Remove from heat and drop in cabbage leaves. Let stand for approximately 2 minutes and then drain. Cut cabbage leaves into julienne strips. In a large mixing bowl, combine vinegar, soy sauce, and sugar. Add cabbage strips and toss. Let stand for 30 minutes in refrigerator or at room temperature. Serve in small individual dishes. Sprinkle with dried red-pepper flakes to taste.

Vegetables
Broccoli with *kimizu*
Serves 4

1   bunch broccoli

Cut broccoli into flowerets with stalks about 3 inches long. Halve the flowerets so that the pieces will be about ½ inch thick at the base. Wash broccoli thoroughly in cold water. Bring 3 to 4 quarts of water to boil in large saucepan. Place broccoli into boiling water, and cook uncovered for about 5 minutes or until just tender. Remove and drain. Serve with *kimizu* sauce.

Kimizu (egg yolk sauce)
Serves 4

2   egg yolks
2   tablespoons water
1   tablespoon rice vinegar
¼   teaspoon salt
¼   teaspoon sugar

Mix all ingredients in the top of a double boiler. Cook slowly over hot water until thick, stirring constantly. Cool quickly by immersing bottom of the double-boiler top in cold water. To avoid formation of skin, keep stirring until cooled to room temperature.

Boiled eggplant
Serves 4

2   medium-size eggplants
       about 2 quarts salted water
1   cup *dashi 1* or *dashi 2*
1⅓   tablespoons sugar
2   tablespoons *sake* or dry sherry
2   tablespoons soy sauce
2   pieces chili pepper

Remove eggplant stems. Cut into halves lengthwise. Make slits in skin diagonally at ⅛-inch intervals; this makes eggplant easier to cook and eat. Cut each half into 3 or 4 pieces, and soak in salted water for several hours to remove bitter taste. Mix *dashi 1* or *dashi 2*, sugar, *sake*, soy sauce, and chili pepper, and bring to boil. Add drained eggplants and cover. Bring to boil and simmer for about 30 minutes, turning once to make sure all pieces are cooked evenly. Serve warm or cold.

String beans with sesame sauce
Serves 4

½   pound string beans, washed and
       with strings removed
       about 3 quarts boiling salted water

SAUCE:

2   tablespoons roasted sesame seeds
½   tablespoon sugar
2   teaspoons soy sauce

Boil string beans in salted water until tender but still crispy. Cut into 1-inch lengths. Prepare sauce by grinding roasted sesame seeds in mortar until creamy. Mix with sugar and soy sauce. Add string beans to sauce and mix well. Let stand for about 30 minutes before serving.

Spinach with lemon sauce
Serves 4

16   fresh, young spinach plants
     (including leaves, stems, and crown
     where root descends)

SAUCE:

1½   teaspoons soy sauce
1   tablespoon lemon juice
1   teaspoon sugar
1   teaspoon *mirin* or cream sherry

Wash and clean spinach. Cook in a covered pot in small amount of boiling water until barely tender. Drain and cool slightly. Cut spinach plants into 1½-inch lengths.

SAUCE: Make sauce by combining soy sauce, lemon juice, sugar, and *mirin*.
     Add spinach, and toss. Serve at room temperature.

NOTE: When fully grown spinach leaves are used, parboil them in plenty of water and cool immediately under running water. This process will help to eliminate the bitter taste.

Green beans with ginger
Serves 4

¼ pound fresh green beans (whole frozen beans may be used)
1 teaspoon finely grated fresh gingerroot
1 teaspoon soy sauce

Wash fresh green beans and remove ends. Put water in a saucepan and bring to a boil. Reduce heat and add beans. Boil uncovered until just barely tender, still crunchy, and green (about 5 to 10 minutes). Drain and rinse in cold water to stop cooking. Cut beans into 2-inch pieces. For each serving, place 18 to 20 beans in small dish. Sprinkle each serving with ¼ teaspoon finely grated fresh gingerroot and ¼ teaspoon soy sauce.

Whole simmered okra pods
Serves 4

1 pound 2- to 3-inch-long young okra pods
1⅔ cups water
4 tablespoons soy sauce
4 tablespoons *sake* or dry sherry
1 teaspoon sugar

Wash okra and cut off stems. Mix water, soy sauce, *sake,* and sugar in saucepan. Bring to a boil. Drop okra into the boiling water, cover, and reduce heat. Simmer about 5 minutes or until just tender. Serve hot in individual dishes sprinkled with cooking sauce.

Sushi and *Sashimi*

Sushi rice
Serves 4

NOTE: The key to *sushi* preparation is *sushi* rice. Once the rice is ready, you can serve it with almost any kind of topping.

1 ¼	cups short-grain rice, thoroughly washed and drained
1 ½	cups water
¼	cup white vinegar
1	tablespoon sugar
½	teaspoon salt
1 ½	tablespoons *sake* or dry sherry

Bring water to boil in a heavy saucepan. Add rice and cover. Simmer until water has been absorbed; this should take about 15 minutes. Turn off heat and let rice sit for another 15 minutes. In a small bowl, mix together vinegar, sugar, salt, and *sake.* Stir into rice. Mix gently but thoroughly, trying not to mash the grains. Cover and let rest for 15 minutes. *Sushi* rice is ready for topping.

Sushi cucumber bars
24 Bars

2	cucumbers
1	teaspoon *wasabi* (Japanese

horseradish) paste or prepared
mustard
sushi rice

Line bottom of 8-inch square pan with waxed paper. Wash
and peel cucumbers, and slice thinly into lengthwise strips.
Remove ends of each strip so it measures about 4 inches.
Make a layer of cucumber strips on the bottom of the pan.
Overlap if necessary. Spread with *wasabi* paste or mustard.
Spoon on *sushi* rice and spread evenly. Cut an 8-inch square
of waxed paper and place over rice. Put another 8-inch square
pan on top of waxed paper. Press down firmly. Place a weight
in top pan. Let pans stand for 1 to 1½ hours.

TO SERVE: Remove weight and top pan. Remove waxed
paper. Invert rice-cucumber onto cutting board. Peel off
waxed paper. With a sharp knife, cut into squares approximately 1½ inches in size. (Wipe knife with wet cloth each
time to facilitate cutting.)

Sashimi (sliced raw fish)
Serves 6

1½	pounds sea bass, tuna, or other similar fish (bones removed)
3	cups shredded lettuce, cabbage, cucumber, or *daikon* (or radishes or turnips)

SAUCE:

1	teaspoon dry *wasabi* (Japanese horseradish) or dry mustard mixed with 1 teaspoon hot water

OR

 1 teaspoon freshly grated gingerroot
½ cup soy sauce

Remove skin and any dark portion from the fish. Using a long, very sharp knife, slice fish on an angle into pieces about 1½ inches wide and ½ inch thick. Chill fish and vegetables until ready to serve. Place shredded vegetables in a shallow dish and arrange pieces of sliced fish so they overlap each other. Mix *wasabi* or mustard paste or grated gingerroot with soy sauce and serve in a small bowl. The sliced fish is dipped into this sauce while being eaten.

NOTE: A variety of fish may be used for this recipe: saltwater flatfish like sea bass, tuna, or swordfish. Shrimp and prawns also make delicious *sashimi*. Regardless of the kind of fish or seafood used, it must be as fresh as possible.

Tofu Dishes

Hiya-yakko (cold *tofu* dish)
Serves 4

 4 4-ounce pieces silky *tofu*
¼ cup soy sauce
1½ tablespoons *mirin,* sweet white
 wine, or cream sherry
¼ cup *dashi 1*

GARNISHES:

radish flowerets
watercress leaves

RELISH:

    (1) mustard paste (prepared with powdered mustard and water), *wasabi* (Japanese horseradish) paste, or grated gingerroot

    (2) chopped scallions (including green stalks)

Keep fresh *tofu* in water for several hours, changing water occasionally. Bring mixture of soy sauce, *mirin*, and *dashi 1*, to boil and let cool to room temperature. Cut *tofu* into 1-inch cubes and float them in ice water to serve. Decorate with garnishes. Serve with sauce and relish of your choice.

NOTE: Individuals can dip pieces of *tofu* in a small bowl of sauce to which relish is added.

Cooked *tofu*
Serves 4

3   cups *dashi 1* or *dashi 2*
3   tablespoons soy sauce
1   tablespoon *sake* or dry sherry
2   teaspoons sugar
3   4-ounce pieces *tofu*, each cut into 4 squares
1   medium-size onion, halved and sliced
4   Chinese mushrooms, soaked in water to soften, with hard stems removed, and cut into bite-size pieces
1   small carrot, peeled and sliced

2 scallion stalks, cut into 1-inch
lengths

Bring mixture of *dashi 1* or *dashi 2*, soy sauce, *sake*, and sugar to boil. Add vegetables (except scallions) and boil for 2 to 3 minutes. Gently add *tofu* pieces and let simmer another 4 to 5 minutes. Add scallions just before removing from heat. Serve hot.

Tofu snack
Serves 4

1 4-ounce cake *tofu*, sliced in half
horizontally and vertically
1 tablespoon vegetable oil
1½ tablespoons soy sauce
1 tablespoon toasted sesame seeds
1 scallion, thinly sliced, including
green stalk

Rinse *tofu* and let dry between paper towels for about 20 minutes. Cut drained *tofu* into triangles to form 8 equal pieces. Heat oil in a skillet and add half the *tofu*. Pan-fry a few seconds until golden, then flip pieces over and fry other sides. Remove *tofu* with slotted spatula to a serving dish. Repeat with rest of *tofu*. Pour soy sauce over fried *tofu*. Sprinkle with sesame seeds and scallion slices. Serve immediately.

Fruit Dishes

Oranges with wine
Serves 4

2 large oranges, peeled and cut into
¼-inch slices

4   tablespoons red wine
2   teaspoons sugar

Mix all ingredients in a salad bowl and let stand for several hours in refrigerator. Serve chilled.

Pears poached in white wine
Serves 4

4   firm ripe cooking pears
¾   pint white wine
½   cup sugar
2   tablespoons lemon juice
20   coriander seeds

Peel pears and cut into halves. Bring mixture of white wine, sugar, lemon juice, and coriander seeds to boil in enameled pan and add pear halves in one layer. Let simmer for about 15 minutes. Remove from heat and let pears cool in juice. Serve cold with a tablespoon of juice per serving.

Beef Dishes

Beef *Teriyaki*
Serves 4 to 5

½   tablespoon juice of gingerroot (grate a chunk of gingerroot and squeeze juice)
1   clove garlic, grated or pressed
¼   cup soy sauce
1   tablespoon *mirin,* white port, or sweet white wine
1   pound flank steak

Mix gingerroot juice, garlic, and soy sauce together with *mirin*. Marinate beef in the mixture for 30 to 60 minutes. Drain marinade and reserve. Broil beef over high heat according to preference. Boil and skim off reserved marinade to serve as sauce. Slice broiled beef into ¼- to ⅙-inch thickness to serve.

Sautéed vegetables with veal
Serves 4

1	tablespoon soy sauce
1	tablespoon *sake* or dry sherry
½	pound lean veal, shredded into small julienne strips
2	teaspoons sesame oil
1	small carrot, cut into julienne strips
2	dried Chinese mushrooms, soaked in water to soften and cut into thin slices
4	ounches canned bamboo shoots, cut into julienne strips
½	pound bean sprouts, washed and drained well
	salt and pepper to taste
2	scallion stems, cut into julienne strips

Sprinkle soy sauce and *sake* over shredded veal, and mix. Heat sesame oil and sauté veal until it changes color evenly. Add carrot, Chinese mushrooms, and bamboo shoots, and continue cooking, stirring constantly. Add bean sprouts when carrots become wilted. Season with salt and pepper. Continue stirring. When bean sprouts become somewhat trans-

parent, stir in scallions, and cook another 2 to 3 minutes.
Serve hot wrapped with Japanese thin omelet (see page 141).

Shabu-shabu (beef and vegetables in broth)
Serves 6

1½	pounds boneless sirloin steak, sliced very thin and cut into 2-inch pieces
2	medium zucchini, washed and cut into ½-inch cubes
6	carrots, scraped, cut into narrow lengthwise strips 2 inches long, and parboiled
6	scallions, including green stalks, cut into narrow, lengthwise 2-inch strips
1	can bamboo shoots, sliced
4	ounces *tofu*, drained, washed, cut into ½-inch cubes
12	small fresh white mushrooms
6	ounces *kishimen* (flat, broad noodles), cooked, drained, and cut into 3-inch lengths
6	cups chicken broth

PONZU SAUCE:

¾	cup soy sauce
½	cup fresh lemon juice

Arrange steak, zucchini, carrots, scallions, bamboo shoots, *tofu*, mushrooms, and noodles in rows on a large platter or tray.

PONZU SAUCE: Combine ingredients and serve in small individual bowls.

Bring chicken broth to a near boil in an electric skillet or fondue pot placed in the center of the dining table. As the broth simmers, each individual diner picks out a piece of beef or vegetable or *tofu* from the large platter and with fondue fork or chopsticks swishes it around until it is ready to eat. To the Japanese the swishing sounds like *shabu-shabu*. After removing the food from the broth, the diner dips it into the *ponzu* sauce bowls and eats it.

Seafood Dishes

Barbecued seafood
Serves 4

2	tablespoons *sake*, wine or dry sherry
¼	teaspoon salt
8	big shrimp, head and shell removed, and deveined
4	ounces fillet of flounder, cut into 8 squares
	pepper to taste
8	medium-size mushrooms, washed and trimmed
½	large green pepper, cut into 8 squares
8	cherry tomatoes
	salt and pepper to taste
2	tablespoons lemon juice
8	long skewers

Sprinkle salt and white wine over shrimp and flounder pieces. Sprinkle with pepper. Let stand for about 30 minutes. On each skewer, thread a mushroom, a shrimp, a piece of green pepper, a piece of flounder, and a cherry tomato. Turning the skewers occasionally, grill or broil over medium to high heat for about 10 minutes or until fish and shrimp are cooked. Sprinkle with salt, pepper, and lemon juice while hot and serve.

Crab-stuffed cucumbers
Serves 6 or 8

NOTE: This dish can be served as an hors d'oeuvre or as the first course for dinner.

      2   ounces crab meat, cooked or canned
      2   tablespoons *mirin* or cream sherry
      2   medium-size cucumbers
           salt
      1   cup water
      2   strips sweet red pepper
     12   sprigs watercress

Flake crab meat and combine with 1 tablespoon *mirin*. Set aside. Peel cucumbers, sprinkle with salt, and let marinate for 10 minutes. Wash off salt. Cut one end off cucumber and scoop out seeds. Boil 1 cup of water. Put watercress in and cook for 2 minutes. Drain. Plunge into cold water and then squeeze dry.

Place 3 sprigs of cress and 1 strip of red pepper inside the hollowed-out cucumber. Then stuff crab meat mixture around cress, using chopstick or end of spoon. Slice into 1/2-inch disks. Place disks on serving dish and sprinkle with remaining *mirin*.

Tempura (featuring shrimp)
Serves 4

1   dozen large shrimp
     various fresh vegetables of your
     choice (for example, 8 snow-pea
     pods, 4 mushrooms, 1 small
     zucchini)
     cooking oil

BATTER:

1   egg
     ice-cold water to make up to 1 cup
     along with egg
1   cup sifted flour

SAUCE:

¼   cup *shoyu*
1   cup *dashi 2*
¼   cup *mirin* or 1½ teaspoons sugar

CONDIMENTS:

     dish of freshly grated *daikon* (or
     radishes)
     dish of freshly grated horseradish

OR

dish of freshly grated gingerroot

Shell shrimp, leaving tail fins attached. Remove black veins. Slit undersection to prevent excessive curling. Wash shrimp and dry thoroughly. Wash vegetables, dry thoroughly, and cut into pieces about the same length as shrimp.

BATTER: Combine egg with ice-cold water in mixing bowl. Sift in flour and stir lightly with wooden spoon or chopsticks. Batter should be thin. Use right away.

Fill deep saucepan or deep-fat fryer at least three-quarters full of cooking oil and heat until very hot. Dip shrimp and vegetables one at a time into batter. Drop food pieces coated with batter into hot oil. Cook vegetables first. Large bubbles will form. When bubbles become small, *tempura* is done. Drain and serve hot with warmed sauce.

SAUCE AND CONDIMENTS: Mix *shoyu, dashi,* and *mirin* in a casserole and boil several minutes. Serve sauce in separate bowls together with separate condiment dishes of *daikon* (or radish), and gingerroot or horseradish. The diner stirs as much of each condiment as he or she chooses into the bowl of sauce. The diner dips the hot *tempura* into sauce-condiment mixture and eats it.

Fish Dishes

Fish baked in foil
Serves 4

8   mushrooms, trimmed and sliced
1   medium-size onion, sliced in rings
1   small carrot, peeled and sliced
4   3½-ounce pieces fresh salmon
4   teaspoons *sake* or dry sherry
    salt and pepper to taste
4   lemon wedges
4   sheets of aluminum foil, each
    about 12 by 15 inches

Preheat oven to 400°F. Place several slices of carrot and mushroom, and onion rings in the center of each piece of foil. Arrange a piece of salmon on top of vegetables on each foil sheet. Cover fish with rest of vegetables and sprinkle with salt, pepper, and dry sherry. Close foil pieces tightly so that no liquid or vapor escapes. Bake in hot oven for 15 minutes. Serve hot with lemon wedges.

Shioyaki (salt-broiled fish)
Serves 4

4   small cleaned trout with head and
    tail
    salt
4   lemon wedges

Wash fish and pat dry. Make some incisions in the skin; this will permit the seasoning to penetrate and also prevent skin from breaking. Sprinkle salt over both sides of fish and let stand for 30 minutes. Broil or grill about 4 minutes on one side, then turn and broil the other side for an additional 5 to 6 minutes, or until skin is crisp.

If fish are grilled, threading them onto skewers will make turning them over easier and keep them from curling—3 small oiled metal skewers or 3 wet bamboo skewers should be inserted through each fish. Serve hot with garnish of lemon wedges.

NOTE: You can substitute any white-fleshed fish such as rockfish or mackerel. If a larger fish is filleted, be sure that the skin is left on for broiling.

Nitsuke of fish (boiled fish in seasoned stock)
Serves 4

4   5-ounce slices (pieces) white-fleshed fish (sea bream, sea bass, or flounder, and so forth), bones and skin intact

½   cup *dashi 1*

½   cup soy sauce

⅓   cup *mirin,* white port, or sweet white wine

1   chunk (thumb size) gingerroot, cut into needles for garnish

Make some incisions in skin of fish pieces. In a shallow flat pan large enough to place fish in one layer, bring mixture of *dashi,* soy sauce, and *mirin* to boil. Place pieces of fish carefully in one layer while sauce is boiling. Cover and cook for 5 to 7 minutes, basting fish occasionally with sauce, until fish is done. Serve hot in a deep plate with generous amount of cooking liquid and sprinkle ginger needles over top.

Teriyaki (featuring salmon)
Serves 6

1½   pounds filleted salmon, cut into 6 pieces

SAUCE:

3   tablespoons *mirin,* sweet sherry, or white port

3 tablespoons chicken stock, fresh or canned
½ cup soy sauce

GLAZE:

¼ cup *teriyaki* sauce (see above)
2 tablespoons chicken stock
1 tablespoon sugar
1 teaspoon cornstarch dissolved in 1 tablespoon water

PREPARE SAUCE: Combine *mirin,* soy sauce and stock, in bowl. Set aside ¼ cup. Place salmon fillets in sauce and marinate for about 30 minutes.

PREPARE GLAZE: Combine *teriyaki* sauce, chicken stock, and sugar in saucepan. Bring almost to boil, then reduce heat. Stir cornstarch and water mixture into sauce. Stir constantly while cooking until glaze becomes somewhat thickened and syrupy.

Preheat broiler. Drain excess sauce from fillets and broil 4 to 5 minutes on one side, basting with sauce. Turn fillets. Baste, broil 5 minutes more. When fillets are browned lightly and flake easily, remove from broiler. Spoon warm glaze over each serving.

Chicken Dishes

Steamed chicken
Serves 4

2 boneless chicken breasts (young), skin removed

    1   tablespoon salt
    2   tablespoon *sake* or dry sherry

    SAUCE:

    3   tablespoons soy sauce
    1   tablespoon lemon juice
    1   tablespoon *dashi 1*

    GARNISH:

    shredded raw vegetables, like
    cabbage, carrots, iceberg lettuce,
    etc.

Sprinkle salt over chicken breasts and let stand for 15 minutes. Then quickly wash chicken under cold water to remove excess salt. Pat dry with paper towel. Place chicken in a deep dish to fit inside a steamer. Sprinkle meat with *sake*. Cover dish with aluminum foil. Steam over vigorously boiling water in closed steamer for 15 minutes, or until meat is cooked through. Let cool to room temperature. Slice into ¼-inch pieces. Serve garnished with shredded raw vegetables. Mix soy sauce, lemon juice, and *dashi 1*, and serve separately in small dish.

Broiled Chicken Livers
Serves 4

    3   tablespoons *sake*
    1   tablespoon soy sauce
    1   teaspoon sugar
    1   1-inch piece fresh gingerroot,
        grated
    8   chicken livers, trimmed of fat
        freshly ground black pepper
    4   small skewers

Combine *sake,* soy sauce, sugar, and sliced gingerroot in a mixing bowl. Add chicken livers, stirring and turning them so they are covered with sauce. Marinate overnight in refrigerator. Remove chicken livers from marinade and cut each liver in half. Reserve marinade.

Preheat broiler. On each of 4 small skewers, string 4 chicken-liver halves. Place skewered livers under broiler about 4 inches from heat and cook 5 minutes. Brush with remaining marinade, turn, and broil on the other side for 4 to 5 minutes, or until no longer pink. Serve on skewers, sprinkled with freshly ground black pepper.

Umani (vegetables with chicken)
Serves 6 to 8

2	whole boneless chicken breasts
2	cups chicken stock, fresh or canned
1/4	cup *shoyu*
2	tablespoons sugar
2	cups bamboo shoots, cut into about 3/4-inch cubes
2	cups fresh mushrooms, washed and trimmed; cut in half if large
2	cups canned water chestnuts, drained
2	medium carrots, peeled and cut into about 3/4-inch cubes
1/2	cup chopped scallions
1	cup fresh string beans (frozen beans can be used), cut into 1-inch lengths

Cut chicken breasts into pieces approximately 1 inch wide and 2 inches long. Bring chicken stock to a boil. Add chicken, *shoyu,* sugar, bamboo shoots, mushrooms, water chestnuts, carrots, and scallions. Simmer covered over low heat 15 to 20 minutes, or until chicken and vegetables are just tender. If using fresh string beans, cook them in separate pot in boiling water for 5 minutes, or until just tender. Drain and add to cooked chicken and vegetable mixture. Serve hot.

Yakitori (featuring chicken)
Serves 4

2   boned whole chicken breasts or 4 boned legs, cut into 1½-inch chunks
6   scallions, including green stalk, cut into 1½-inch strips
8   bamboo skewers
    freshly ground black pepper

SAUCE:

½   cup soy sauce
2   tablespoons lemon juice
2   tablespoons *mirin* or sweet sherry
    sugar to taste

SAUCE: Combine sauce ingredients in a bowl.

Place chicken chunks and scallion strips alternately on 8 skewers. There should be 3 strips of scallion and 3 chunks of chicken on each skewer. Brush with sauce. Broil on one side about 5 minutes; brush again with sauce and broil on the other side 5 minutes, or until lightly brown. Boil remaining sauce for 1 or 2 minutes.

TO SERVE: Place 2 skewers of chicken chunks and scallion strips on plate. Sprinkle with freshly ground black pepper and moisten with small amount of remaining sauce.

Egg Dishes

Chawanmushi (steamed egg dish)
Serves 4

3	eggs
2	cups *dashi 1* (or chicken stock)
1	teaspoon soy sauce
½	teaspoon salt
1	boneless chicken breast, cut into 8 bite-size pieces (or 8 bite-size pieces of pork)
4	small shrimp (or 4 small pieces fish fillet)
	a pinch of salt
2	teaspoons *sake*
4	button mushrooms
4	half-slices bamboo shoots (or 4 water chestnuts)
2	ounces parboiled spinach, cut in 1-inch lengths

NOTE: *Chawanmushi* is eaten out of special *chawan* (teacup) bowls, ceramic vessels with removable lids. If not available, use large coffee or custard cups, tightly covered with aluminum foil. Keep covered until ready to eat.

Beat eggs in bowl. Add *dashi 1* or stock seasoned with soy sauce and salt. Put mixture through fine strainer to blend whites and yolks of eggs thoroughly. Sprinkle salt and *sake* over chicken, shrimp, and mix. Let sit for 10 minutes. In each of four *chawan* bowls place one shrimp, one mushroom, two pieces of chicken, and one piece of bamboo shoot. Fill the bowls with egg mixture up to ½ inch from the rims. Place a few spinach leaves in each bowl and cover. In a steamer large enough to hold four bowls, bring water to boil. Set bowls in the steaming pot, cover, and steam about 13 to 15 minutes over medium heat. To test for readiness, pierce surface of custard with toothpick. When juices do not run out of hole, *chawanmushi* is ready. Serve in bowls.

Spinach cake
Serves 6

1½	pounds cooked spinach
4	eggs, beaten
1	cup low-fat unsweetened yogurt
3½	ounces bread crumbs
	salt, pepper, and nutmeg to taste
1	tablespoon butter or margarine

Butter a 9-inch pie dish. Heat oven to moderate temperature. Squeeze as much water as possible out of spinach and cut into about ½-inch pieces. Mix together beaten eggs, yogurt, bread crumbs, and spinach, and season with salt, pepper, and nutmeg. Put mixture in buttered pie dish and bake 45 minutes, or until cooked through.

Japanese thin omelet
Serves 2

4	eggs
	vegetable oil
	dash of salt
	dash of sugar (optional)

Beat eggs. Add sugar and salt if desired. Lightly brush with oil the bottom and sides of an omelet pan or a frying pan. Heat pan over moderately high heat. When a drop of water sprinkled on pan surface evaporates instantly, pour enough egg mixture to cover bottom of pan evenly. Tilt pan over heat, coating entire surface with egg mixture. When outer edges of omelet are cooked, center will be done. Remove pan from heat and gently turn omelet over, using spatula. Cook reverse side of omelet until dry and set. Remove omelet from pan and place on serving dish.

Repeat procedure until all egg mixture has been used. Omelets may be cooled and then cut in any desired shape. Garnish with parsley, grated white turnip, or any other item you wish.

NOTE: This omelet is often shredded and served as a garnish for rice or salad. You can also use this omelet to wrap *sushi* rice or to roll up sautéed vegetables.

Chapter 11

EAT WELL AND STAY TRIM THE JAPANESE WAY

One day on ABC-TV's *Good Morning America* program, Linda Evans, the glamorous star of television's nighttime soap opera *Dynasty,* began talking about her diet and her own special recipe for keeping in trim. She thought that her health and good looks came from her "terrific metabolism," and this, in turn, she attributed to her good eating habits.

She said that she always sat down to dinner in anticipation of eating something with pleasure.

"Set the table," she said, "put out the candles, light the fireplace, make the setting attractive to yourself. Prepare something you really like, take small portions, take twenty minutes or more to eat it." Then, she went on, "You're full, you're content, you feel good about yourself, and you're happy."

Although she did not mention the Japanese way of dining, without realizing it, Linda was discussing several of its main and most important features:

- "Set the table," she said, "put out the candles, light the fireplace, make the setting attractive to yourself." As you can see, she was simply expounding the principal means the Japanese use to make the dining area conducive to calmness and good appetite. "Half the battle," she might have said, "is in getting the right atmosphere for a good meal."

- "Prepare something you really like," she went on. Once again, the Japanese do not believe in eating anything that is unappetizing, overcooked, or not fresh. They always select the best foods and clean them well before any further preparation.
- "Take small portions," she continued. This is strictly a Japanese habit. Eating a variety of foods and eating less of each serving is a way of life—a way of life that has paid off in their being much less overweight than Americans.
- "Take twenty minutes or more to eat it," she said. Unconsciously, Linda was expounding the Japanese way—slow, calm, easy—of eating. Food assimilated slowly tends to fill the stomach more fully and signals satisfaction more quickly to the brain than food bolted down in haste. It is another key element in eating the Japanese way.
- And in conclusion, Linda said, "You're full, you're content, you feel good about yourself, and you're happy." That's the aim of any good Japanese meal.

The five main points Linda Evans made inadvertently about Japanese cooking and eating can be an excellent basis for a proper American diet. Of course, she covered none of the actual foods prepared, cooked, and eaten, but she did cover most of the other salient points about Tokyo cuisine.

GOING JAPANESE THE AMERICAN WAY

The point of this book is not to influence you into throwing away all your pastry pans and roasting ovens to cook only on a hibachi and substitute noodles and rice for bread and butter. The point is to make you *think* about food selection and preparation done the Japanese way. Sure, you can whip up a good Japanese meal every once in a while— use some of the foods suggested here and cook them in the way described—but you don't need to go totally Japanese and never enjoy a hamburger or french fries again.

If you did that, you'd be liable to make the same mistakes the Japanese do in their diet—adding too much salt, for example. No, the thing to do is to adapt the measures that make the Japanese diet a slimming one, one that keeps you fighting weight, puts your body in a healthful and trim condition.

Following the Japanese way will cut down your fat intake to about 30 percent of your daily Calories. In the process, it will reduce the amount of saturated fat you eat that causes cholesterol deposits, and you'll get the proper amount of "good" carbohydrates and fibers in your diet.

Let's take the groups of food one by one.

Fish, Meat, and Poultry

Although for a long time the Japanese menu did not include meat and poultry, it does now. However, these are eaten with a definite Japanese philosophy of moderation in mind. The Japanese go easy on meat and poultry, concentrating on fish. Frankly, no one needs red meat at every meal;

that's an American tradition, dating from the early days when every man wanted to eat the diet of the rich and affluent.

If you cut down on your meat consumption and substitute vegetable sources, you can get protein with little fat and no cholesterol. Out of the long list of meats and poultry, choose chicken, turkey, and fish if you can. They contain a lot less total fat and less saturated fat than beef and pork, for example.

Another Japanese trick: Always keep portions small. In the United States today most people who watch their weight try to keep their meat intake to about three to four ounces per serving—quite a comedown from the days when the average recipe called for a half-pound of meat per person!

Incidentally, in many cookbooks still on the bookshelves, recipes call for eight to twelve ounces of meat per serving! Take a look. You'll be surprised. In the same books, the Calorie count (added later on) is usually for a meat portion that is 3½ or 4 ounces.

Because the Japanese include many different dishes in a meal—or they can if they want to—one dish may contain only an ounce of food or even less. Remember to keep your meat, fish, and poultry intake *down*. It'll pay off in fewer pounds on your frame.

HOW TO SELECT WEIGHT-CONSCIOUS MEAT CUTS

In choosing meat cuts, think Japanese. Buy as lean as possible. For beef that means eye of round, shoulder, rump, chuck, and sirloin-tip roasts; flank, round, tenderloin, and sirloin-tip steaks; dried and chipped beef; extra-lean ground beef; lean stew meat. Forget pork. For lamb select the leg, shoulder or rib chop, and loin chop.

For poultry choose chicken (broilers and fryers), turkey, and Cornish game hens.

Generally, fish are low in fat and saturated fat—except for tuna canned in oil, salmon, fresh or canned, sardines canned in oil, and mackerel. Most shellfish are high in cholesterol, but are low in fat and serve as good substitutes for meat. Shrimp, a favorite with the Japanese, is higher in cholesterol than other shellfish.

HOW TO PREPARE WEIGHT-CONSCIOUS FOODS

In preparing meat, fish, or poultry, think Japanese. Trim off all the fat you can before cooking. Be sure to get rid of all the fat the butcher wraps around the roast. Also watch out for the large amount of fat *under the skin of poultry.*

When roasting meat, apply vegetable oil on the top. Baste meat with pan juices. Roast at a low temperature; you'll get rid of more fat that way. Putting the roast on a rack lets the fat drip off.

Broil or roast fish, meats, and poultry. Even though the Japanese do a lot of frying, keep yours to a minimum. If you do fry, be sure to apply only a light amount of fat to the meat or fish, and allow it to cook for a short time only, keeping down the amount of oil absorbed.

You can borrow another trick from the Japanese by poaching fish with water flavored with lemon juice, vinegar, or *sake,* and other herbs and spices. Or you can poach fish in a typical clear-soup mix.

HOW TO GARNISH IN A WEIGHT-CONSCIOUS WAY

The Japanese avoid gravies entirely probably because they have always used more fish than meat or poultry and do not savor gravies. You can forget about thick sauces, too. Remember the Japanese like to prepare food as close to the natural state as possible before serving. Although they use condiments and seasonings, they do not like them to over-power the original flavor of the food or in any way alter its natural taste.

Milk and Buttermilk

The Japanese use very few dairy products of any kind. However, there is no need for you to eschew all milk, cheese, or eggs. In fact, the Japanese *do* use eggs today as we do.

You can always limit your servings of milk to two a day. Eight ounces of milk or an ounce of hard cheese is considered one serving. Many overweight people who diet switch to low-fat or skim milk. If you do, you'll be getting less cholesterol as well as less fat. Note that homogenized milk has 3.5 percent butterfat. By substituting low-fat milk, you can cut down to 2 percent butterfat and then on down to 1 percent butterfat.

Incidentally, buttermilk is low-fat milk; use it in baking or making pancakes. Yogurt made with partially skimmed milk contains about 1 percent butterfat. Use milk or milk powder in your coffee. Light cream has 20 percent butterfat; heavy whipping cream, 38 percent butterfat. Whipping-cream substitutes, artificial sour cream, and fake cream cheese are made with coconut oil, which has a lot of saturated fat in it. Avoid them.

Cheeses and Eggs

Cut down on hard and processed cheeses; they are high in fat and cholesterol. Use low-fat cheese slices or cottage cheese. Regular creamed cottage cheese has 4 percent butterfat; low-fat cottage cheese has half that amount or less. Forget cream cheese; it has 37 percent butterfat!

As for eggs, the yolk of a single egg contains almost an

entire day's serving of cholesterol. You don't need to eat eggs every day, anyway. When you do, separate the yolk from the white. You can eat as many egg whites as you want; they are a low-calorie source of protein.

In a recipe that calls for one or two eggs, substitute two egg whites for one whole egg, or three egg whites for two whole eggs. If you are used to eating noodles made from eggs, try to find some made from substitutes like rice or vegetables.

Fats and Oils

When you must cook with fats or oils, cook Japanese. Don't use saturated animal fats like butter, lard, suet, salt pork, or chicken fat, especially if your blood cholesterol level tends to be high. Use vegetable cooking oils, but avoid solid vegetable shortening. Instead, be sure you use polyunsaturated vegetable oils and margarines. Some margarines are almost as saturated in fat as butter; the softer the margarine, the less saturated it is. Margarine should contain twice as much unsaturated fat as saturated fat. On the package, the letter "P" stands for polyunsaturated fat, and "S" stands for saturated fat. The "P/S" ratio should be two to one or higher.

Like the Japanese, make use of sesame oil, which has a nutty flavor and is perfect for salads and for sautéing vegetables. Safflower oil is mild and also good for making your own mayonnaise. Corn oil is excellent for baking. Soybean and peanut oils are strong and can be blended with other oils.

NOTE: Learn to check out the ingredients list on all processed foods. If a vegetable-oil product contains coconut or palm oil, leave it alone. These two vegetable oils are the only ones that are heavy in saturated fat.

Avoid eating commercial baked goods; they are probably cooked with saturated fat.

In baking recipes replace melted shortening or butter with vegetable oil. Make your own salad dressings, using polyunsaturated vegetable oil, mayonnaise-type salad dressing, yogurt, or buttermilk. You can even make an herb dressing, with vinegar or lemon juice but without any oil; that's doing it the Japanese way.

When frying or sautéing, go light on the vegetable oil. Just brushing the pan, or using a nonstick spray-on oil, is enough.

Vegetables and Fruits

The message is a simple one:

Do as the Japanese do. Eat plenty of vegetables and some fruit.

And in the case of vegetables, cook them lightly and quickly, using as little seasoning or condiments as possible.

Desserts

Although the Japanese do eat small sweet pastries, they do not always eat them for dessert. A piece of fresh fruit usually suffices as dessert, and if a small pastry is served, it is probably *very* small.

Pastries and cakes may be familiar to the Japanese diner, but pie is not. If you want to eat the Japanese way, you don't have to *forget* cakes and pies and pastries—not at all!—but when you eat them, do so as the Japanese would if they had them: small pieces, please!

Remember this: The smaller the piece, the more fulfilling the dessert.

Forget chocolate candies and icings of all kinds. A lot of chocolate candies are made with cream or have coconut centers.

Condiments and Snacks

Some nuts and seeds—for example, sunflower and sesame seeds—are all right to eat because they contain a high proportion of polyunsaturated fat and no cholesterol. Nevertheless, they are high in total fat and in Calories. So don't consume them to excess.

The best nuts—at least, from a standpoint of the type of fat involved—are walnuts, pecans, almonds, and peanuts.

But watch out for peanut butter! It is high in total fat, *and* in Calories. You can substitute peanut butter for meat, but eat it only infrequently. Use only two tablespoons for an equivalent meat serving. Old-fashioned peanut butter is better than the processed kind. The processing uses hydrogenated oil to keep the peanut butter from separating. Also, some brands use sugar and salt in their manufacture. In any case, stay away from nuts served as a snack while you are on a diet to lose weight, because their fat contents are anywhere between 45 and 75 percent of their weight.

Eating Out

When you dine out, you don't have to go to a Japanese restaurant to eat the Japanese way. Simply watch what you select. Choose dishes that avoid heavy sauces and condiments and gravies; select those that are served as close to the natural state as possible. Also, avoid cheeses, fried foods, pot pies, and the like.

- *For appetizers:* Choose fresh fruits and vegetables or juices. Seafood cocktails are good. However, avoid seasoned butter or oils, and sour or sweet cream.
- *For soups:* Select clear consommé or broth with noodles or vegetables. However, avoid

onion soup, egg soup, creamed soup, and cheese flavorings.

- *For salads:* Choose green and tossed salads. A chef salad can include chicken, turkey, seafood, tuna, lean roast beef, lean ham. Select clear gelatin molds. Choose cole slaw or potato salad—*if* they have a minimum of mayonnaise. However, avoid cheese and cream dressings.
- *For fish:* Choose any variety prepared without fat. Avoid tartar sauce.
- *For poultry:* Select chicken, turkey, Cornish game hen, prepared without fat and with the skin removed. However, avoid goose, duck, and fried or batter-dipped coatings.
- *For red meat:* Always select lean hind-quarter cuts of beef, lamb, and pork. You can choose any kind of veal except for flank cut. But avoid prime cuts, gravies, breaded coatings, and any ground beef.
- *For fruit:* You don't need to be very strict about them. However, avoid cream or whipped toppings.
- *For vegetables:* Eat as many plain vegetables as you like. Be sure beans and peas come without oil or sauce.
- *For bread:* Choose any sandwich bread, breadsticks, hard rolls, French and Italian breads, wafers, and toasts. However, avoid biscuits, croissants, corn muffins, bran muffins, blueberry muffins, and butter rolls.
- *For desserts:* Choose angel-food cake, gelatin desserts, frozen fruit ices, and low-fat dairy products. But avoid ice cream and nondairy milk substitutes.

SAYONARA TO FAT!

- *For beverages:* Drink low-fat milk products, artificially sweetened carbonated beverages, fruit juices, coffee, and tea. However, avoid cream and nondairy milk substitutes.
- *For condiments:* Choose pickles, relishes, mustard, steak sauce, catsup, lemon juice, vinegar, spices, and herbs.

Many restaurants use animal fats or saturated vegetable fats to prepare dishes. If you are dining in an Oriental restaurant, you can eat fried foods, since the Japanese and Chinese use soybean oils—which contain unsaturated fat—for frying. But be aware of the fact that these oils contain as many Calories as animal fats do.

As a general rule of thumb, think Japanese:

- Go for the dish that is simply prepared and served.
- Go for the dish that does not have any fat in it.
- Concentrate on poultry, fish, and seafood—just as the Japanese do.
- You can always order your fish broiled without butter.
- You can even ask for salad dressing on the side so you can add whatever amount you want yourself.
- Ask for oil or vinegar for your salad dressing, which you can apply yourself.
- You can even order your meat and potatoes served without gravy or sauce.

As Linda Evans said: "You're full, you're content, you feel good about yourself, and you're happy."

What more could you ask?

Nanimo! Nothing!

Chapter 12

LOSE UP TO FIFTEEN POUNDS IN A MONTH

If you are overweight and want to lose pounds, you must remember that you cannot do so without making a serious and sustained effort. Yet, simply by being aware of your weight problem you have taken one giant step toward control because that awareness has made you conscious that you are eating too much.

Dieting is a matter of pushing consciousness one step farther and converting it into action. You must use much more thought and care than before in your choice of food, your daily menu, and the way you eat your food, and you must adhere to that regimen in a steadfast manner.

If you are one of those people who start dieting by eating carrot sticks and a cup of yogurt at the table while the rest of the family eats steak and potatoes, you are in for a rude awakening. Fasting can help you lose body weight dramatically, but you are not only depriving yourself of the nutrients necessary for the normal functioning of your body, but you are cheating yourself of the physiological and psychological satisfactions of eating—including sitting at the table and sharing a convival meal with your loved ones.

SAYONARA TO FAT!

Weight control is a long-lasting, serious project, including the loss of weight and the maintenance of that weight loss afterward. It must be worked out scientifically and logically, taking into consideration your eating habits and those of everyone around you. It requires more attention and skill to plan a "diet meal" than a regular meal.

Even with the most skillful planning, you may experience frustration; physical and psychological exhaustion may sap your strength before you attain your desired weight. You may find a way to balance the physical suffering you experience from the restricted intake and the lack of variety in your menu with the mental fulfillment you get from your eventual achievement of a substantial weight loss.

FIFTEEN-DAY MENUS TO SHED FIFTEEN POUNDS

There are fifteen-day sample menus in this chapter that can help you lose up to fifteen pounds in a month—eating in the Japanese manner. As you can see at a glance, it is not very difficult to eat to lose weight as long as you cut down on fats and oils. The problem of sugar per se is actually less serious. Never forget, however, that practically all sweets (cookies, cakes, and other desserts) contain butter, fat, or cream—*in addition to sugar.* Fruit salads and compotes are the only desserts that are exceptions to this rule.

Here are some helpful weight-losing hints for you to ponder while you are on your diet:

The heavier you are to begin with, the faster you lose weight while adhering to any given diet.

For example, if you are 35 percent overweight, you may lose fifteen pounds in a month on the diet given here, but if you are only 20 percent overweight, you may not lose more than eight pounds.

Do not expect to see any weight loss after being on a diet only one day.

The body somehow tends to resist losing weight. You may see no change in weight for two or three days. Any "diet" that claims to lose several pounds on the first day usually involves only a loss of bodily fluids—which is not true weight loss, since the pounds return once you drink fluids again.

Do not be disappointed when you find that you are slightly heavier one day than you were the day before.

Body weight can fluctuate one or even two pounds from day to day, depending on your physical condition. It is the overall weight change in one week, rather than in one day, that makes the vital difference.

When you eat meat, buy it as red as possible and trim off as much fat as you can before cooking.

As has been emphasized in this book all along, one of the main reasons Japanese cuisine is light and good for weight control is that it includes many low-fat animal-protein sources like fish and shellfish, and that most fat from any red meat is trimmed off during preparation.

Limit the preparation of food that requires additional fat or oil.

Use cooking methods like grilling, broiling, steaming, and boiling in a stock.

Do not prepare more food than you can eat. Throw away all extras if you happen to prepare too much.

This is not a carte-blanche injunction to waste food. It is only a reminder that any excess must be dealt with either in an easy way or a hard way: from the table to the garbage can (easy to get rid of), or from the table to the unnecessary fat around your stomach (hard to get rid of). Make your choice: Get rid of that excess now—or pay for it later.

SAYONARA TO FAT!

Try to prepare food for several people rather than for only one.

It is easier to prepare a 3½-ounce slice of roast beef for several people than grill a 3½-ounce steak for one. You can achieve more variety in your diet when you prepare for a group. You need 1 teaspoon of oil to sauté 4 ounces of spinach, for example, but you need only 2 teaspoons of oil to prepare a pound of spinach for four people

Keep the amount of salt and spices you eat to a minimum.

When a dish is salty, you need to eat more potatoes, bread, or pasta to compensate. In addition, spicy food tends to *increase* your appetite.

If there is any sauce remaining on the plate after you eat, leave it—don't sop it up!

Sauce often contains fat or oil.

Eat regularly. Avoid skipping meals or nibbling on snacks between meals.

In snacking, you will find it very difficult to keep track of the amount of food you eat. Snack food tends to be high in Calories. Skipping a meal breaks your bodily rhythm and causes unnecessary fatigue. Missing a meal often causes you to eat more than necessary when you sit down to your next meal.

Do not eat food that is high in Calories just before going to bed.

If you ingest Calories that will not be used for energy right away, they will be converted to body fat and stored . . . unattractively.

These are only a few pointers that are directly related to practicing weight control. There are, of course, many important points to keep in mind for healthy living—physical and mental—as have been discussed throughout this book.

The actual menus given here have been developed to help you lose weight, not to maintain that desired weight once you attain it. To maintain a desired weight, you can usually add another slice of bread for breakfast, exchange low-fat milk or yogurt for natural products, drink a glass of wine or one apéritif for dinner, and put a teaspoon of sugar in your coffee or tea. You may even add a scoop of sherbet to either a lunch menu or a dinner menu.

We hope that you succeed in losing weight while enjoying the diet!

NOTE: An asterisk indicates that the recipe for the item is available in Chapter 10. The measure to the right of the item is the prescribed portion for maintenance of a weight-loss program.

Day 1

Breakfast

tomato juice   *6 fluid ounces*
whole wheat bread   *1 slice*
with butter or margarine   *¼ ounce*
poached egg   *1*
coffee or tea

Morning snack

low-fat milk   *6 fluid ounces*

Lunch

cottage cheese salad with
low-fat cottage cheese   *2 ounces*
carrots, shredded   *1 ounce*
cucumbers, sliced   *2 ounces*
beets, sliced   *2 ounces*
lettuce   *2 to 3 leaves*
seasoned with salt, pepper,
lemon juice, and salad oil   *1 teaspoon*
whole wheat crackers   *4 to 5*
tea, coffee, or diet drink

Afternoon snack

apple   *1*

Dinner

hiya-yakko* (cold *tofu*)
silky *tofu*   *4 ounces*
served with a sauce   *2 tablespoons*
spinach *sunomono**
*umani** with
young lean chicken meat   *2 ounces*
bamboo shoots   *¼ cup*
mushrooms   *¼ cup*
water chestnuts   *¼ cup*
carrot   *¼ medium*
string beans   *⅛ cup*
prawn and cucumber soup* with
prawns   *1⅓ ounces*
cucumber   *⅙*
mushroom   *1 piece*
plain boiled rice   *4 ounces cooked*
canned pineapple in its own juice   *1 slice*
tea

Day 2

Breakfast

grapefruit ½
cornflakes *1 ounce*
with low-fat milk *6 fluid ounces*
and honey *1 teaspoon*
coffee or tea

Morning snack

low-fat unsweetened yogurt with *6 ounces*
fruit jam of your choice *1 teaspoon*

Lunch

Japanese noodle soup* with
soba (buckwheat noodle) *2 ounces (dry)*
chicken breast (skin removed) *2 ounces*
scallions *½ ounce*
*dashi** or chicken broth *8 fluid ounces*
apple ½

tea

Afternoon snack

diet drink
vegetable sticks
(carrots, celery, cucumber) *1 ounce each*
whole wheat crackers *4 to 5*

Dinner

beef consommé   *6 fluid ounces*
with julienne of celery, carrots, scallions   *½ ounce each*
barbecued seafood* with
shrimp   *2 large*
flounder   *1 ounce*
mushrooms   *2*
green pepper   *⅛ large*
cherry tomatoes   *2*
lemon   *⅛*
rice boiled in chicken broth   *4 ounces cooked*
green salad   *2 ounces*
with oil   *1 teaspoon*
vinegar or lemon juice
orange with wine*   *1 portion*
tea

Day 3

Breakfast

cantaloupe ½
puffed wheat *1 ounce*
with low-fat milk *6 fluid ounces*
and honey *1 teaspoon*
coffee or tea

Morning snack

banana *1 medium size*

Lunch

sliced turkey breast *2 ounces*
with tomato ½
green pepper, sliced ¼
radish *5 pieces*
lettuce *2 to 3 leaves*
lemon juice
rye bread *1 slice*
diet drink

Afternoon snack

low-fat milk *6 fluid ounces*

Dinner

cucumber and sesame-seed salad* with
cucumber   1/3 *small*
sesame seeds   1 *teaspoon*
crab meat   1/6 *cup*

Japanese thin omelet* (2 layers)
egg   1

sautéed vegetables with veal*
lean veal   2 *ounces*
bean sprouts   2 *ounces*
carrot   1/2 *ounce*
Chinese mushroom   1/2 *piece*
bamboo shoots   1 *ounce*
scallions   1/2 *stalk*
sesame oil   1/2 *teaspoon*

miso soup*   6 *fluid ounces*
with *miso*
zucchini sliced   1 *ounce*

plain boiled rice   4 *ounces cooked*

fresh peach   1
tea

Day 4

Breakfast

tomato juice   6 *fluid ounces*
puffed wheat   1 *ounce*
with low-fat milk   6 *fluid ounces*
honey   1 *teaspoon*
coffee or tea

Morning coffee break

coffee or tea
graham crackers   2 *(1 ounce)*

Lunch

salad with
avocado, sliced   ¼
boiled shrimp   2 *ounces*
tomato, sliced   ½
lemon juice
whole wheat crackers   5
low-fat milk   6 *fluid ounces*
coffee or tea

Afternoon snack

orange   1

Dinner

steamed chicken* with
young chicken breast *3 ounces*
iceberg lettuce, shredded *1 ounce*
radishes *3*
carrot *namasu** with
daikon (radish) *1 ⅓ ounces*
carrot *⅙*
boiled eggplant* with
eggplant *½*
clear soup* *6 fluid ounces*
with hard-boiled egg *½*
boiled spinach *½ ounce*
plain boiled rice *4 ounces cooked*
canned fruit salad (water packed) *3 ounces*
tea

Day 5

Breakfast

shredded wheat   *1 ounce*
with low-fat milk   *6 fluid ounces*
honey   *1 teaspoon*
coffee or tea

Morning snack

fresh pear   *1 medium size*

Lunch

Belgian endive (witloof chicory)   *2 ounces*
with Swiss cheese, diced   *1 ounce*
apple, diced   *½*
walnuts, coarsely chopped   *1 tablespoon*
oil   *1 teaspoon*
vinegar
lettuce   *2 to 3 leaves*
whole wheat crackers   *5*
coffee or tea

Afternoon snack

ice milk   *2 ounces*

Dinner

daikon salad with shrimp*
daikon (radish) ⅙
cucumber, cubed *1 tablespoon*
shrimp, diced *1 large*
beef *teriyaki** with
flank steak *3½ ounces*
sautéed watercress *3 ounces*
miso soup* with
miso (bean paste) *1 tablespoon*
tofu *1 ounce*
dashi 1 or *dashi* 2* *6 fluid ounces*
scallions, sliced *1 teaspoon*
plain boiled rice *4 ounces cooked*
assorted fresh fruit
kiwi ½
pineapple *1 slice*
cherries 7
tea

Day 6

Breakfast

grapefruit   ½
whole wheat bread   *1 slice*
with butter or margarine   ¼ *ounce*
low-fat milk   *6 fluid ounces*
coffee or tea

Morning snack

apple   ½

Lunch

herring (brine packed)   *1 fillet*
with boiled potato, sliced   *3 ounces*
string beans, boiled   *1 ounce*
cucumber, sliced   *2 ounces*
tomato, sliced   ¼
lemon juice
coffee or tea

Afternoon snack

diet drink or coffee or tea
saltine crackers   *5*

Dinner

boiled asparagus   *3 large*
with lemon juice
roast leg of lamb (well trimmed)   *3½-ounce slice*
boiled green peas   *3 ounces*
with carrot, diced   *1 ounce*
onion, diced   *1 ounce*
butter or margarine   *¼ ounce*
dinner roll   *1*
fresh pear   *½*
coffee or tea

Day 7 (Note: This Is a Sunday Special)

Brunch

grapefruit *½*
pancakes (made with low-fat milk) *2, 4 inches in diameter*
with maple syrup *1 tablespoon*
coffee or tea

Midday snack

low-fat unsweetened yogurt *6 ounces*
with honey *1 teaspoon*
apple *½*

Dinner

*chawanmushi** (steamed egg dish) with
egg *¾*
chicken meat *¼ breast*
shrimp *1 small*
vegetables in the recipe *1 portion*
Chinese cabbage in vinegar* *¾ leaf*
*nitsuke** (fish cooked in stock) with
white-meat fish *5 ounces, bones included*
string beans *2 ounces*
with sesame sauce* *½ tablespoon*
plain boiled rice *4 ounces cooked*
strawberries *3½ ounces*
with sugar *1 teaspoon*
tea

Day 8

Breakfast

grapefruit ½
grilled-cheese bread or toasted bread with cheese
whole wheat bread *1 slice*
low-fat processed cheese *1 slice*
coffee or tea

Morning snack

low-fat milk *6 fluid ounces*

Lunch

tomato juice *6 fluid ounces*
open sandwich with
rye bread *1 slice*
lean roast beef *2 ounces*
onion, sliced *1 slice*
tomato, sliced ½
lettuce *2 to 3 leaves*
prepared mustard
coffee or tea

Afternoon snack

low-fat unsweetened yogurt *6 ounces*
with honey *1 teaspoon*

Dinner

egg drop soup*
with chicken broth   6 *fluid ounces*
egg   ½
teriyaki of salmon*   *4-ounce piece*
daikon (radish), grated   2 *ounces*
whole simmered okra pods*   2 *ounces*
plain boiled rice   4 *ounces cooked*
fresh peach   *1*
tea

Day 9

Breakfast

vegetable juice   *6 fluid ounces*
whole wheat bread   *1 slice*
with butter or margarine   *¼ ounce*
poached egg   *1*
coffee or tea

Morning snack

low-fat milk   *6 fluid ounces*

Lunch

clear soup*   *6 fluid ounces*
with boiled spinach or crown daisy   *2 ounces*
broiled chicken livers*   *1 skewer*
broiled leek   *3 1-inch pieces*
with mushrooms   *2 pieces*
on a skewer (seasoned with salt and lemon juice)
plain boiled rice   *4 ounces cooked*
tea

Afternoon snack

orange   *1*

Dinner

chicken noodle soup   *6 fluid ounces*
with fine noodles   *1 tablespoon*
stuffed cabbage with
cabbage   *2 leaves*
lean ground beef   *3 ounces*
onion, chopped   *½ ounce*
parsley, chopped   *1 teaspoon*
oil or butter   *1 teaspoon*
watercress salad   *2 ounces*
with oil   *1 teaspoon*
lemon juice or vinegar
canned pear in its own juice   *3½ ounces*
coffee or tea

Day 10

Breakfast

grapefruit   ½
whole wheat bread   *1 slice*
with butter or margarine   *¼ ounce*
boiled egg   *1*
coffee or tea

Morning snack

low-fat milk   *6 fluid ounces*

Lunch

salad with
canned tuna (water packed)   *2 ounces*
boiled potato, sliced   *2 ounces*
tomato wedge   ½
lettuce   *2 to 3 leaves*
oil   *1 teaspoon*
lemon juice   *½ teaspoon*
rye bread   *1 slice*
coffee or tea

Afternoon snack

low-fat unsweetened yogurt   *6 ounces*
with honey   *1 teaspoon*

Dinner

crab-stuffed cucumber* with
cucumber   *2 ounces*
crab meat   *⅓ ounce*
*shabu-shabu** with
beef (lean slices)   *3½ ounces*
zucchini   *2 ounces*
scallions   *1 ounce*
bamboo shoots   *2 ounces*
carrots   *1 ounce*
tofu   *1 ounce*
mushrooms   *2 pieces*
Japanese dry noodles   *1 ounce*
chicken broth   *1 cup*
ponzu dipping sauce*   *3 tablespoons*
fruit salad with
orange   ¼
apple   ¼
banana   ⅓
cherries   7
sweet liqueur   *1 tablespoon*
tea

Day 11

Breakfast

vegetable juice *6 fluid ounces*
shredded wheat *1 ounce*
with low-fat milk *6 fluid ounces*
honey *1 teaspoon*
coffee or tea

Morning snack

pear *medium size*

Lunch

salad with
canned sardine in tomato sauce *3 pieces*
fresh tomato, sliced ½
cucumber, sliced *2 ounces*
celery sticks *1 ounce*
lemon juice or vinegar
whole wheat bread *1 slice*
coffee or tea

Afternoon snack

low-fat milk *6 fluid ounces*
graham crackers *2*

Dinner

spinach cake*   *1 portion*
steamed mussels   *8 ounces in shells*
with onion, minced   ¼ *onion*
thyme
green salad   *2 ounces*
with oil   *1 teaspoon*
lemon juice or vinegar
canned peach in natural juice   *3 ounces*
coffee or tea

Day 12

Breakfast

grapefruit ½
puffed wheat *1 ounce*
with low-fat milk *6 fluid ounces*
honey *1 teaspoon*

Morning snack

low-fat milk *6 fluid ounces*

Lunch

stuffed tomato *1 large*
with boiled ham, diced *1 ounce*
celery, chopped *½ stalk*
cucumber, diced *1 ounce*
mayonnaise *½ tablespoon*
lettuce *2 to 3 leaves*
rye bread *1 slice*
coffee or tea

Afternoon snack

diet drink
boiled egg *1*
celery and carrot sticks *1 ounce of each*

Dinner

beef consommé   *6 fluid ounces*
with parsley, chopped   *1 teaspoon*
fish baked in foil* with
salmon   *3½-ounce piece*
fresh mushrooms   *2 pieces*
onion   *2 slices*
carrot   *3 to 4 slices*
lemon wedge   *1*
boiled potatoes with parsley   *3 ounces*
green salad   *2 ounces*
with oil, lemon juice, or vinegar   *1 teaspoon*
grapes   *3½ ounces*
coffee or tea

Day 13

Breakfast

grapefruit ½
puffed wheat *1 ounce*
with low-fat milk *6 fluid ounces*
and honey *1 teaspoon*
coffee or tea

Morning snack

apple ½

Lunch

clear soup* *6 fluid ounces*
with diced *tofu,* *1 ounce*
sliced scallion *1 teaspoon*
*sashimi** with
sea bass *3 ounces*
shredded *daikon* *1 ounce*
wasabi paste with soy sauce *1 tablespoon*
green beans with ginger* *2 ounces*
plain boiled rice *4 ounces cooked*
tea

Afternoon snack

low-fat milk *6 fluid ounces*

Dinner

tomato aspic with
tomato juice, spiced   *½ cup*
sliced green olives   *1 teaspoon*
diced celery   *1 tablespoon*
diced cucumber   *1 tablespoon*
served with mayonnaise   *1 teaspoon*
grilled minute steak (flank steak)   *3½ ounces*
mashed potato prepared   *3 ounces*
with low-fat milk   *1 tablespoon*
and butter or margarine   *1 teaspoon*
boiled broccoli (no butter)   *3 ounces*
with lemon juice
pear poached in wine sauce*   *½ pear*
coffee or tea

Day 14 (Note: This Is a Sunday Special)

Brunch

grapefruit   ½
scrambled egg   *1*
with butter or margarine   ¼ *ounce*
low-fat milk   *1 tablespoon*
bacon (well drained)   *2 strips*
whole wheat bread   *1 slice*
low-fat milk   *6 fluid ounces*
coffee or tea

Midday snack

low-fat milk   *6 fluid ounces*
whole wheat crackers   *5*
fresh peach   *medium size*

Dinner

clear soup with chicken*   *6 fluid ounces*
with chicken breast   ⅛ *chicken breast*
boiled broccoli   *3 ounces*
with *kimizu** (egg yolk sauce)   *1 tablespoon*
shioyaki of trout*   *1 small*
with grated radish   *2 ounces*
a wedge of lemon
cooked *tofu** with
tofu   *3 ounces*
onion   ¼, *small*
Chinese mushroom   *1 piece*

SAYONARA TO FAT!

carrot   ¼, *small*
scallion   ½ *stalk*
plain boiled rice   *4 ounces cooked*
canned fruit salad (water packed)   *3 ounces*
tea

Day 15

Breakfast

orange juice   *3 fluid ounces*
whole wheat bread   *1 slice*
with butter or margarine   *¼ ounce*
boiled egg   *1*
coffee or tea

Morning snack

low-fat milk   *6 fluid ounces*

Lunch

salad with
canned salmon in water   *2 ounces*
tomato, sliced   *½*
canned sweet corn   *2 ounces*
lettuce   *2 to 3 leaves*
lemon juice or vinegar
rye bread   *1 slice*
coffee or tea

Afternoon snack

low-fat unsweetened yogurt   *6 ounces*
with honey   *1 teaspoon*

Dinner

tofu snack*   *1-ounce portion*
*yakitori** (barbecued chicken)   *3 ounces*
with scallions   *1 ounce*
chicken broth   *6 fluid ounces*
with chopped scallions   *1 teaspoon*
spinach with lemon sauce*   *2 ounces*
grapes   *3½ ounces*
tea

GLOSSARY OF JAPANESE CUISINE TERMS

Although each word or phrase in this handy reference for Japanese cookery has already been explained when first introduced in the text, in some cases the same term is used again and again in subsequent passages without accompanying explanation.

To help jog the reader's memory, this Glossary lists each Japanese term with a brief description alongside it.

abura-age: deep-fried *tofu* puffs

aemono: one of the basic types of salad; the word means "mixed things"; this type of salad is usually with thick sauce

agemono: a type of cooking involving frying in vegetable oil

aka: means red (see *akami, aka-miso*)

akagai: the ark-shell clam; also called pepitona clam

akami: the Japanese term for the fillet of red meat from tuna fish or beef

aka-miso: a red type of *miso*

ama-ebi: a type of raw shrimp

an: *azuki* jam or sweet *azuki* paste

anago: the conger eel, a saltwater fish

aoyagi: the red clam, similar to the American quahog

atsu-age: deep-fried *tofu* cutlets, cakes, or cubes

GLOSSARY

awabi: the abalone clam

azuki: a small red bean

bancha: a type of Japanese tea

buri: the full-grown yellowtail, or tuna fish, over 35 inches long

cha: tea

chawanmushi: a dish of steamed egg resembling a custard

chazuke: word meaning "tea-soaked"; a way of soaking rice with tea before eating

chikuwa: a fishcake

chirashi (chirashi-zushi): a kind of *sushi* with shredded seafood and vegetable mixed with vinegar and rice

chu: medium (see *chu toro*)

chu-miso: golden-type *miso*

chu-toro: the pinkish meat between the belly and the red meat of the tuna fish

daikon: the Japanese white radish, very long and sold in chunks

daizu: the dried soybean; must be soaked before simmering

dashi: a basic soup and cooking stock often made from dried bonito flakes and kelp

date maki: an omelet containing ground fish, often served as a *sushi* delicacy

donburi: a ceramic serving and eating bowl that is large and deep; it often comes with a lid to fit, keeping warm liquids hot *donburimono:* a type of dish served in *donburi* bowls; usually rice with a side dish placed on top of the rice

ebi: shrimp

edamame: young green soybeans

endo: the green pea

enokitake: a slender white mushroom

fuki: coltsfoot

furikake: a commercial seasoning made from dried bonito, seaweed, sesame seeds, sugar, salt, and MSG

ganmo (ganmodoki): deep-fried *tofu* burger

gari: ginger pickled in vinegar, eaten with *sushi*

genmaicha: a type of Japanese tea with roasted rice grains

ginnan: ginkgo nuts

gobo: burdock root

gohan: a serving of rice that is cooked and ready to eat, or a Japanese meal

gohanmono: a type of dish with a rice base

goma: sesame seeds; white seeds are used in most recipes and for eating, black seeds are used for garnish

gyokuro: a type of Japanese tea

hakusai: Chinese cabbage, a long variety up to 16 inches in length

hamachi: the year-old yellowtail, about 30 to 35 inches long

hamaguri: the Pismo Beach clam

hasu: the lotus root

GLOSSARY

hijiki: dried sea vegetation that resembles licorice in appearance

hiya-yakko: a type of cold *tofu* dish

hojicha: a type of roasted Japanese tea

ichiban dashi: a type of Japanese cooking stock used mostly for clear soup

ika: the squid

ikura: salted salmon roe

inada: the baby yellowtail

inari-zushi: a kind of *sushi,* with vinegared rice put inside a fried bag of *tofu*

kabayaki: a type of dish, grilled eel with thick sauce

kabocha: a type of squash

kaibashira: a large scallop; also called *tairagai*

kaki: the oyster

kama: a special pot for cooking rice

kamaboko: cakes made out of fish paste

kamado: traditional Japanese cooking fireplace

kamasu: the barracuda

kani: the crab, usually used as crab meat

kappa maki: a *sushi* dish featuring cucumber

kara-age: a type of frying in which ingredients are lightly dusted with cornstarch before being fried in vegetable oil

kasuzuke: a type of pickle prepared in *sake* lees

katsuo: the bonito

katsuobushi: bonito flakes, used in *dashi* and in other recipes

kikurage: a type of mushroom, tree ear, or elephant ear

kimizu: a type of egg sauce

kinugoshi-tofu: silky *tofu*

kishimen: broad, flat noodles

kobashira: a small scallop

koi: the carp

koji: a mixture of rice, barley, or soybeans used for making soy sauce, *miso,* etc.

kojizuke: a type of pickle prepared in *koji*

kombu: dried, cultivated kelp or sea vegetation or sea tangle; also spelled *konbu*

kome: rice, as a grain or as a crop; see *gohan*

konro: grill similar to Western barbecue grill

koya-dofu: freeze-dried *tofu*

kuikiri: one of the styles of serving a formal Japanese meal

kuromame: the black bean

kyuri: the cucumber

maguro: the name for the tuna family

masu: the trout

matcha: a type of Japanese green tea, powdered

menrui: the generic name for the entire family of noodles

meshimono: the same as *gohanmono*

GLOSSARY

mirin: a sweet, syrupy rice wine, related to *sake;* used for cooking

mirugai: the horseneck clam, or geoduck

miso: fermented soybean paste

misoshiru: soybean paste soup, a rather thick type of soup

misozuke: a type of Japanese pickle prepared in *miso*

mizutaki: a one-pot dish often featuring simmered (boiled) chicken

mochi: a type of rice cake mainly eaten during the New Year period

momen-tofu: regular *tofu* (bean curd)

moyashi: the bean sprout

mushimono: steamed foodstuffs, including vegetables, meats, eggs, fish, and shellfish

nabe: the word for cooking pot or saucepan

nabemono: one-pot cooking at the dining table

nama-age: the same as *atsu-age*

namasu: a type of salad

nasubi: the eggplant

natto: a type of condiment made with fermented soybeans

negi: a type of long onion

niban dashi: a type of Japanese cooking stock used mostly for cooking vegetables and for *misoshiru*

nigiri (nigiri-zushi): a vinegared rice-and-fish *sushi* "sandwich" *nimono:* a cooking technique; refers to boiling in a seasoned liquid

ninjin: carrots

nitsuke: term for boiled fish in stock

nori: laver, a type of sea vegetation

norimaki-zushi: sushi featuring dried laver

nuka: rice bran; it is used in pickling to add crispness and flavor to vegetables

nukamiso-zuke: a type of Japanese pickle prepared in rice bran

odori: a word meaning "dance"; it refers to the eating of live shrimp in *sashimi* dining

o-kara: lees left after obtaining soybean milk for making *tofu*

o-kazu: a general term for a side dish

ponzu: originally, the juice of a type of citrus fruit; now a kind of sauce

rakkyo: a type of shallot (scallion) pickled in vinegar

renkon: the lotus root; also called *hasu;* popular vegetable for deep frying and boiling

sake: the salmon

sake: rice wine, the most popular of Japanese alcoholic beverages; also called *nihon shu*

sakekasu: lees left after the production of *sake*

sasa maki zushi: sushi prepared in bamboo leaves

sashimi: the serving of raw fish, thinly sliced, as an appetizer or as a dish

GLOSSARY

sato imo: a field or country potato; called "taro potato"

satsuma imo: the sweet potato

saya-endo: snow peas

senbei: a general term for Japanese cookies

sencha: a type of Japanese tea

shabu-shabu: a kind of one-pot saucepan dish in which the diners cook their own food to each one's taste

shichimi-togarashi: a seven-flavored spice often served with noodle dishes

shiitake: a kind of mushroom

shioyaki: the word for salt-broiling

shiro: the word for white (see *shiro maguro*)

shiro maguro: the word for albacore

shiro-miso: sweet white *miso*

shirumono: general term used for soup course

shoga: fresh ginger, also known as gingerroot; one of the most widely used condiments in Japan

shojin ryori: the cookery of the Buddhists; usually refers to an all-vegetable cuisine

shoyu: soy sauce

shungiku: the garland chrysanthemum, also called "chop-suey greens" and crown daisy

soba: the buckwheat noodle

somen: a type of fine noodle made with wheat flour

su: vinegar made from rice

sudako: boiled octopus served with vinegared soy sauce

suimono: a clear soup

sukiyaki: a type of one-pot dish of simmered beef and vegetables cooked at the table

sumashi (sumashi jiru): the same as *suimono*

sunomono: the term used for a vinegared salad

sushi: an appetizer or dish featuring vinegared rice with various foodstuffs

tai: the sea bream (a fish)

tairagai: a large scallop; also called *kaibashira*

takenoko: bamboo shoots

tako: the octopus

tamago yaki: an omelet, often sweet

tamari: a type of Japanese seasoning obtained from *miso*

tara: the codfish

tare: a type of sauce usually used for broiling fish or meat

tataki: a type of preparation of raw fish, typically bonito and horse mackerel

tekka maki: a thin rolled *sushi* dish featuring tuna

temaki-zushi: a *sushi* offering served wrapped in a cone shape

tempura: a popular dish of deep-fried shrimp; but word describes other deep-fried ingredients

tengusa: a red seaweed

teppanyaki: grilled meat and chicken on a metal plate

teriyaki: a dish of broiled marinated foodstuffs

tofu: soybean curd; high in protein, rich in minerals and vitamins, and low in saturated fats and Calories

torigai: the cockle

toro: the belly of the tuna, used in ordering *sushi* and *sashimi*

tsuke-dashi: a type of light sauce usually served with noodles

tsukemono: "soaked things," referring to vegetables pickled in any of various pickling agents

udo: a fennellike Japanese vegetable usually eaten raw but sometimes used as a garnish

udon: a type of noodle made with wheat flour

umani: a type of dish cooked in sweet cooking stock

umeboshi: a pickled plum

unadon: a kind of *donburimono* featuring grilled eel *(kabayaki)*

unagi: freshwater eel

uni: the sea urchin

wakame: a type of sea vegetation

wakashi: the baby yellowtail

wakegi: scallions

warasa: the baby yellowtail (see *wakashi* and *inada*)

wasabi: a type of green horseradish; powdered *wasabi* is a mustard-type condiment in Japan

yaki-dofu: grilled *tofu*

yakimono: a word used to describe grilled or broiled foods *yakitori:* a word referring mainly to chicken placed on skewers and grilled over charcoal

yama imo: the mountain yam

yokan: a jellylike sweet made from beans

yosenabe: a "gathering of everything" in a stew, including vegetables, fish, *tofu,* and *dashi,* cooked in one pot at the table

zoni: a type of dish served during the New Year period

INDEX

INDEX

INDEX

vegetables *(continued)*
  soup stock, 110
  and veal, 128
vinegar, 29, 38, 51, 83, 99
  and spinach salad, 117
  and *sushi*, 83–86

wakame, 80
wakashi, 75
wakegi, see scallions
warasa, 75
wasabi, see horseradish
watercress, 124, 131
weight control, 17–18, 87, 146–148
weight loss menus, 159–187

weight loss tips, 154–158
wine, see *mirin;* port wine; *sake;* sherry

yaki-dofu, 69
yakimono cooking, 100
yakitori, 36, 199
yams, 19, 61
  see also potatoes
yellowtail, 75, 86
yosenabe, 97

Zen Buddhist cooking, 31–33, 53
zoni, 51
zucchini, 129, 132